THE SHEPHERD'S CODE

KRISTINA WILDS

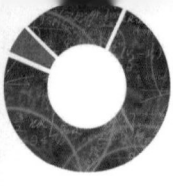
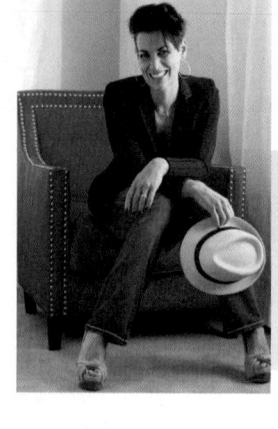

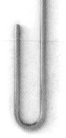

CONGRATULATIONS! You've made a wise decision to invest in your health and well-being.

You've joined a growing group of over 150,000 men, women and children who are discovering the benefits of eating "healing fats"!

The Shepherd's Code (TSC) is a method of healthy eating based on both the most modern science and research available.

TSC is not a fad. It's not a yo-yo or roller coaster diet where you may lose weight for a few weeks only to pack on more pounds later. *The Shepherd's Code System* is a lifestyle change that has the power to dramatically improve your life.

More importantly, *TSC* works 100% of the time. Everyone who follows the simple plan will see results – probably faster than they'd expect. I know this from personal experience. I have also seen the fantastic results achieved by 15 years worth of personal clients.

I receive mountains of correspondence from people who tell me how *TSC* has transformed their bodies and their lives. Like these...

 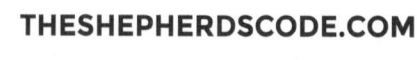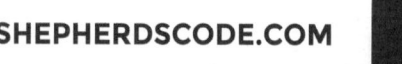

Patty
June 16 at 8:12pm

"I am so excited to announce that **I have now lost 30 lbs in 3 months. This lifestyle is amazing** and I would like to encourage every discouraged person to never give up. If I can do this then anyone can!"

 Brenda - with **Brad**
June 19 at 6:15am

"Here are we before and today pictures. **Between us we have dropped 62 lbs**. Brad is ahead by -2. Brad was in rare form. He was cracking me up with his Grandpa Jones from hee haw act."

 Brenda
June14 at 11:36pm

Today was official weigh in for me. Happy News. **Down a total of 28 lbs, 17 of that since March. BMI is down to 30% with no muscle loss.** I am thrilled, i was losing a lb muscle at every weigh in at the Nutrition Wellness center. This was very encouraging! Hope to post a picture on the weekend.

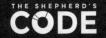

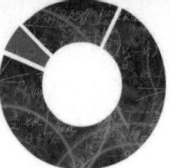

Jesse
June 19 at 6:10pm · · ·

"I'm so glad I found this program I started on April 1 and **was at 268# now down to 233# That is over three bowling balls** that I am not carting around all the time."

👍😍😮

Debbie
June15 at 5:57pm · · ·

"Went to my knee doctor yesterday and I had lost a pound since last week. I am so excited. **That puts me at 24 pounds lost since the middle of March! The best way of life I have ever tried**. I also made the strawberry fat bombs last night and they are wonderful!"

👍😍😮

Donna
June 18 at 6:00pm · · ·

"Next week will be 3 months for me. My goal was to lose 20# the first 3 months. **As of this morning, I have lost 20.5#! Woohoo!**"

👍😍😮

 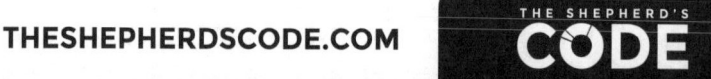

June
June 14 at 3:51pm

"**I am in the fourth day of my third week, and I am down 9 pounds! I must say, I am totally blown away by this new way of eating!** I was so skeptical, because, believe me, I have tried it all! I am also hypothyroid (Graves' Disease) and that has added the extra weight (no pun intended) of trying extra hard to lose because of my (lack of) metabolism. I have been overweight for the last 30 years of my life, and have vowed many many times that this time I am going to do it!"

Colleen
June 13 at 10:49pm

Down a total of 15 pounds in the first 8 days. Wow.

I've received **thousands** of notes just like these. They're pouring in faster than I can read them!

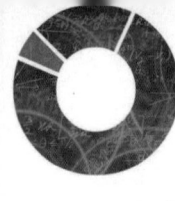

Here's the BOTTOM LINE: If you will make a personal COMMITMENT to follow *The Shepherd's Code System, you will experience the body transformation you desire.* If you're willing to make this COMMITMENT to yourself, then just nod your head in agreement right now as you're reading this.

That simple choice is all it takes to get you started on the road to shedding pounds, shredding fat, increasing your energy and self-confidence, and living an all-around happier and healthier life.

And that's what you want, right?

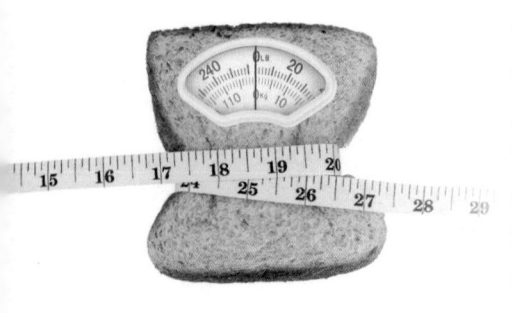

The desire to begin and determination to remain diligent to the *TSC System* will have you on your way to success. I am confident that you will join the ranks of thousands before you who have achieved personal success and transformation.

In as little as a week, I wouldn't be surprised if you start getting second looks and comments from your friends and family about the changes that quickly begin to reveal the new and improved you.

I am excited for you! My guess is you will drop a few dress or pants sizes in the coming weeks. Your life is about to change in a big way, my friend. I can't wait to hear about your success story!

OK. Let's get started...

 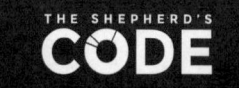

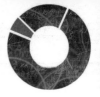

IMPORTANT POINTS TO REMEMBER:

▶ Please follow *TSC* System exactly as it has been laid out for you. Remember, there are scientific reasons for doing things in a certain methodical and specific way. This approach is well documented and backed by scientific and medical journals. Please, do your best to follow the program.

▶ Make sure you are well organized. I recommend using notebooks, notecards, or technological means (cell phones or computers) to keep track of your eating and your progress so you can see the transformation happening in front of your eyes, as well in the cold hard data.

▶ Make sure you access your *The Shepherd's Code* program, bonuses and videos from our member's area. It's simple; first, go here **www.shepcode.com/members**.

▶ Then, enter your email (the same email you used to sign up). There's no password required.

▶ You may want to enlist the help of a supportive friend or family member who can help you stay accountable. I highly recommend you join our *Facebook group* **www.shepcodefamily.com** so you can interact with others in the *The Shepherd's Code* community for support and to learn from their experiences.

▶ Feel free to ask questions on our *Facebook group*. If you still have questions, *please contact our customer support team here* **support@ theshepherdscode.com**

▶ And PLEASE, every time you experience a personal success or breakthrough, *send us an update* **support@theshepherdscode.com** and share it with our *Facebook group*. Your successes will motivate others in the *The Shepherd's Code* community, just as they in return will provide encouragement along your journey.

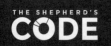

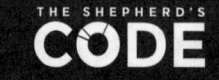

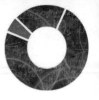

The contents of this document are based upon my opinions of *The Shepherd's Code* unless otherwise noted. This work is intended to share knowledge and information learned through research, experience, and discussions with others. The opinions of others, such as in the comments and the forum, are their own and are not endorsed by *The Shepherd's Code*. The information contained herein is not intended to diagnose, treat, cure or prevent any condition or disease, but rather to provide general information that is intended to be used for educational purposes only. Please consult with your physician or healthcare practitioner if you have any concerns. By using, viewing and interacting with *The Shepherd's Code* or **shepherdscode.com** website, you agree to all terms of engagement, thus assuming complete responsibility for your own actions. The authors and publishers will not claim accountability, nor shall they be held liable for any loss or injury sustained by you. Use, view and interact with these resources at your own risk. All products and information given to you by *The Shepherd's Code* and its related companies are strictly for informational purposes only. While every attempt has been made to verify the accuracy of information provided on our website and within our publications, neither the authors nor the publishers are responsible for assuming liability for possible inaccuracies. The authors and publishers disclaim any responsibility for the inaccuracy of the content, including but not limited to errors or omissions. Loss of property, injury to self or others, and even death could occur as a direct or indirect consequence of the use and application of any content found herein. Please act responsibly. The information provided may need to be downloaded and/or viewed using third party software, such as Acrobat. It's the user's responsibility to install the software necessary to view such information. Any downloads, whether purchased or given for free from our website, related websites or hosting systems are performed at the user's own risk. Although we take great preventative measures, we cannot warranty that our websites are free of corrupting computer codes, viruses or worms. If you are a minor, you can use this service only with permission and guidance from your parents or guardians.

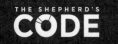

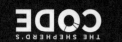
*This book is dedicated
to my dear friend, Elaine;
she was a force.*

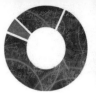

CONTENTS

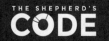

INTRODUCTION

> *"And we know in all things God works for the good of those who love Him, who have been called according to His purpose."*
>
> **Romans 8:28**

> *"Do not be anxious about anything, but in every situation by prayer and petition with Thanksgiving, present your requests to God."*
>
> **Philippians 4:6**

"Your husband has ALS, not Parkinson's," the doctor told me.

The news was devastating. In an instant it effectively reduced the lifespan of my beloved husband, Stan, by ten to twenty years. People like Michael J. Fox could continue living for over twenty years with Parkinson's disease, but ALS was a cruel and painful death that wouldn't afford him that much time.

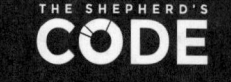

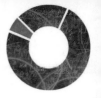

THE SHEPHERD'S CODE

> My husband's illness and death were a tragic, but by the grace of God, these tragedies ended up helping me save my sister's life from the grips of obesity, diabetes, and the potential of a fatal heart attack.

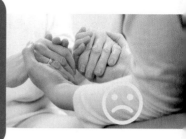

When I learned that Stan was going to die a decade or two earlier than I'd expected, I used the unfortunate opportunity to get stronger rather than weaker. I realized that I was all my five-year-old son Luke had to rely on. So, I began to work out longer and harder. I ate better. I would play the Rocky theme song while driving or getting dressed for the day. I remember thinking, "I can do this. I am strong. It could be worse."

It became clear to me that if Stan could be diagnosed with a deadly, horrible disease just out of the blue, then it very well could happen to anyone I love! It became imperative for me to relay the importance of health and self-care to my family and loved ones! For each of them I encouraged a better eating and exercise regimen.

Little did I know, Stan's illness had changed the course of my destiny.

Years later, I was still encouraging my family to exercise and eat better using a "healing fats" diet. It was then that I found out my sister Kimberly was looking for a way to lose weight and feel better.

When I went to see her, she said, "Wow, you look great! You're glowing and you're so fit. I can see your leg muscles through your jeans!" I felt so thrilled when she complimented me with such sincerity. I said, "Well, I can help you do this too, if you'll trust me."

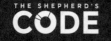

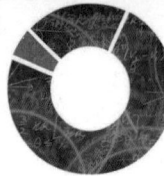

Kimmy was a full-time wife and mother. She had been overweight for at least ten to fifteen years. She was exhausted all the time, chronically in pain with different issues—her back, her shoulder, whatever.

My sister has always been one of the best moms I've known. She does everything with her kids and is extremely involved. But at that time, she needed help. She was the typical example of the person who gives so much of their time and energy to others that they ignore their own needs.

I decided to help her, of course, and she was willing to keep an open mind and hear what I had to say. I explained that first and foremost, she needed to adjust her mindset to the understanding that fats are good for us, not bad.

We have been conditioned by parts of society, as well as the media, to believe that fat is bad. Period. You shouldn't eat real bacon; eat turkey bacon instead. Don't eat butter; margarine is better for you. Those bits of advice are the complete opposite of what we should be hearing and doing for our health. These deceptions hide the fact that fats are very good for you indeed.

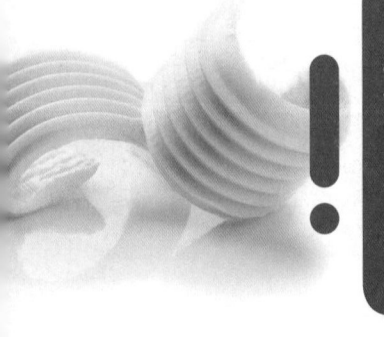

It can be difficult to change a well-in-grained mindset—thinking that fats were unhealthy shaped the diets of an entire generation of people. But we knew less then than we do now. We were misinformed, or led astray, at the least.

> *So you will eat the fat and clothe yourselves with the wool.*
>
> **Ezekiel 34:3**

I can explain to you how divine intervention changed my mind in a minute, but first, let me introduce myself.

My name is Kristina Wilds. I am what's considered a Master Trainer. For the past twenty years, I have worked with individuals who have came to me troubled by being overweight, underweight, and/or disabled. I've been a personal trainer since 1987 and have certifications in Nutrition, Corrective Exercise, Sports Nutrition, Childhood Obesity, and CrossFit.

Since 1987 I have worked as a personal trainer/coach with diverse populations, and have a passion for helping those seeking answers to their health and fitness needs.

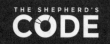

I was married to a man with ALS and served as his primary caregiver. I researched diets, food plans and exercise; everything that one could control, I sought out and researched.

I am proud of my accomplishments, but for a few years, I felt like I was a sham. I had clients paying me to help them lose weight, get in shape, and gain their confidence back. Meanwhile, they had no idea that I was acting like a charlatan. I felt helpless and hopeless.

I had suffered from an eating disorder for many years when I was in my early 20s and 30s, and I have a solid, personal understanding of how food can rule and even destroy your life. I have cried in grocery stores, restaurants, and doctor's offices. I understand the deep frustration because I too tried everything that promised the perfect figure, weight loss, and everything else that I was searching for. I'm also a single mother of a little boy, and I can empathize with people who have busy schedules, time constraints and the craziness of being a mom or dad.

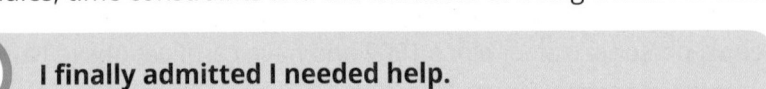 **I finally admitted I needed help.**

I went to a rehab facility to get my life back and learn how to fuel my body properly with real food.

BAM! I was put right into Eating Disorder Boot Camp. The rehab center removed sugar, wheat and flour from my diet. Meals were even weighed! Meal times were set in stone. I ate breakfast at 8 am, lunch at 12 noon, dinner at 5:30 pm and had a metabolic adjustment before bedtime. I followed this schedule for 35 days until I was discharged. I felt amazing and happy that I could eat and actually lose weight!! I was blown away!

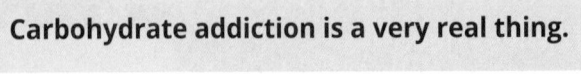 **Carbohydrate addiction is a very real thing.**

 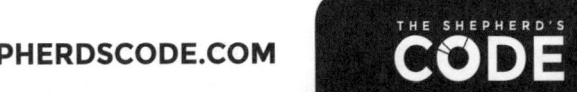

Research has shown that carbs activate certain stimuli in the brain that cause dependence and addiction. There is a phenomenon of craving that occurs in carb/sugar addicts. The craving can be uncontrollable at times and extremely difficult to manage! This craving can lead to binging behavior. There is also withdrawal from carbs and sugar. The withdrawal symptoms include fatigue, irritability and, of course, the intense cravings. (footnote from Boyers, CNHC)

> *You shall have no other gods before me.*
>
> **Exodus 20:3**

I had allowed food, and sugar in particular, to stand in the way of my relationship with God.

It was amazing to finally have the opportunity and courage to show Kimmy, my sister, what I had learned about nutrition. For years I had taken care of myself and clients in this way.

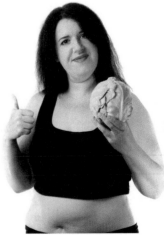

Kimmy listened, and the results she saw were nothing short of miraculous. Once Kimmy adjusted to eating the rich and satisfying fats, like butter, heavy cream, cheese, and bacon, it was easy for her to continue. She started losing two pounds a day, and within two weeks, she dropped 12 pounds, without surgery, diet pills,

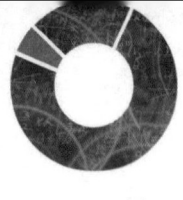
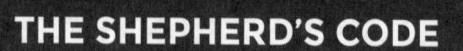
exercise, or even counting a single calorie, all by eating more—specifically, eating more foods that contained "healing fats" and few carbohydrates.

I helped her eliminate the worldly temptations of addictive sugar and genetically modified foods. Those only lead to a life of being overweight, obese, and diseased.

Most important, getting my sister to commit to *The Shepherds Code System* helped to save her life. Now she can spend more time with her family and in fellowship with others.

The results of *TSC* are lasting. Even though my sister travels a lot and dines out frequently, she has been able to stick to the plan!

Her husband is an attorney, and they attend a lot of charity events. Shortly after Kimmy started *TSC*, she took a trip to St. Bart's. During this vacation, while her friends drank and ate chips, she stuck to her food plan and felt great... She thought it was miraculous.

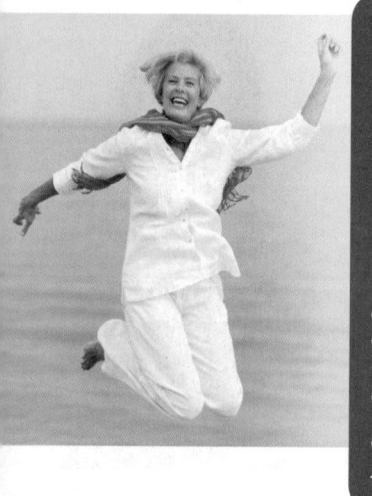

Normally, my sister would have given in to peer pressure, because of FOMO, fear of missing out. She didn't want to feel different or left out. But she was feeling so wonderful and had so much energy. She said, "I'm not going to do that. I'm going to stick to what I need to do for me." She did, and the meals were easy and manageable... and she still had a great time on her trip.

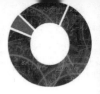

YOU CAN DO IT TOO

THE SHEPHERD'S CODE CAN HELP YOU IF:

You're chronically overweight, tired, and sick, with a deep frustration at having tried so many other plans, pills, and procedures that did not work.

You can't find a diet that will help you to lose weight and improve your overall health and fitness.

You don't think you have the time, the discipline, or even the desire to commit to a new lifestyle.

You're not sure you have enough money to buy healthy food, or you feel guilty or uncomfortable about making an investment of time and money in your diet and health.

You worry that your family will be disappointed or angry if you don't make their favorite unhealthy dishes anymore.

You wonder whether being overweight and unhealthy is simply inevitable because you've been chubby your entire life.

You wonder why you must feel deprived to look great and be healthy.

You pretend that being fat doesn't matter because what's on the inside—your soul—matters more than looks and your health. You may also struggle with feeling worthy enough to invest in a change to something "superficial," like your weight.

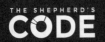

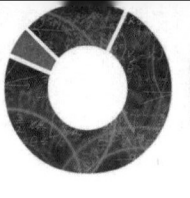

> *Or do you not know that your body is a temple of the Holy Spirit within you, whom you have from God? You are not your own.*
>
> **1 Corinthians 6:19**

Knowing this truth leads to the conviction that I am to treat this body as a vessel of worship by being the best temple of the Holy Spirit I can be. When I don't even protect my body from harmful foods, it's like saying, "I don't care how your temple is treated."

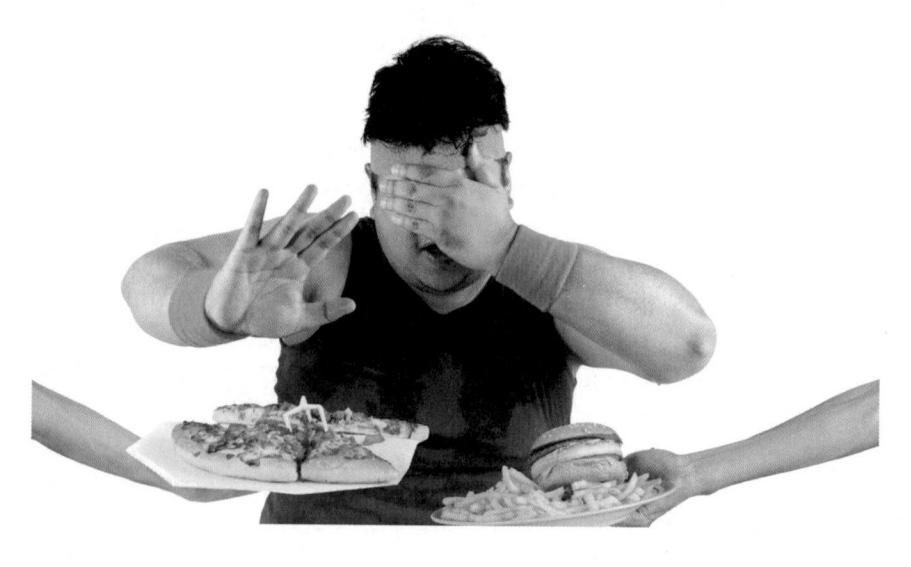

TSC is a step-by-step system that works by eating more fat, in particular, "healing fats", and fewer carbs. Scientific evidence about what to eat is in perfect sync with this food plan and the Bible. This is what makes *The Shepherd's Code System* so different, amazing, and truly life changing.

TSC is a low-carb, very high-fat, moderate-protein food plan that replaces unhealthy carbs with "healing fats". The meals are simple, tasty and easy to prepare, and the snacks are really satisfying.

One reason *TSC System* is so successful is that on it you never go hungry. I can attest to that! Fat is much more satiating than carbs or protein. When the body begins to burn fat, instead of carbs or sugar, you will feel incredible, not to mention, you'll look incredible too.

TSC provides rapid results, which is huge for most people. People like immediate gratification. *TSC* System gives you really fast results, fast enough that it seems like immediate gratification. Life is precious. Don't wait around wasting time!

Diseases such as diabetes, heart disease, dementia, cancer, inflammation, or any kind of autoimmune disease, shorten our precious life on Earth by as much as 10, 20, or even 40 years.

 These chronic and painful diseases can be reduced or eliminated by using *TSC System.*

What I'm about to reveal pierces through the lies propagated by leftist big food corporations that pollute our food supply, marketing GMOs with their addictive sugars and deadly chemicals as healthy. This book uncovers the big pharmaceutical and food industry's billion-dollar deception, which they hope you never discover. They plan to keep you hooked on their drugs, having horrible side effects like weight gain, headaches, irritability, loose stools, rashes, and even death.

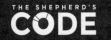

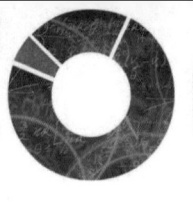

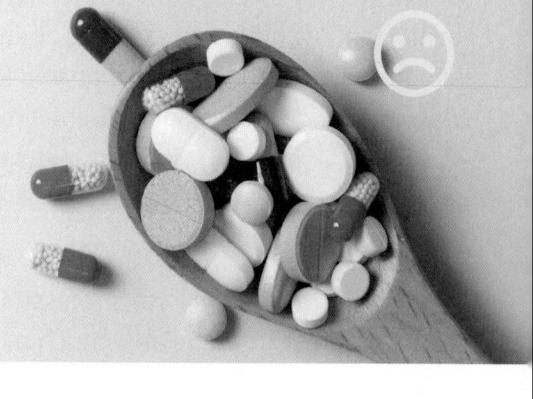

The truth is, *TSC* System also helps remove the need for medications. It's easy, and it doesn't lead to weight gain, or any of those other side effects.

Traveling and dining out are a big part of many people's lives. So it's good to note that even on vacation or out at dinner, you can still stick to *The Shepherd's Code*

My sister is a busy wife and mother who lost weight with minimal effort. She made some changes, and it just fell off. This is evidence that it is possible, even likely, for you to lose weight, just as my sister did.

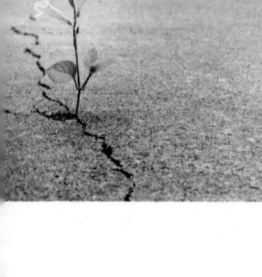

TSC provides hope. It's the scientifically-proven diet plan you need to finally overcome your individual obstacles and get what you really want.

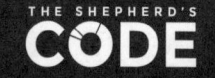

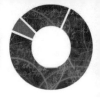

HOW DOES IT WORK?

THE SHEPHERD'S CODE SYSTEM CONSISTS OF 7 SIMPLE STEPS:

Step #1:
Develop a *The Shepherd's Code* Mindset

Step #2:
Free Yourself from Addiction to Sugar

Step #3:
Get Started on the Ideal You

Step #4:
Rest and Eat Right

Step #5:
Resist Temptation

Step #6:
Claim It

Step #7:
Maintain Your Strength
and Dignity for a Lifetime

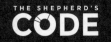

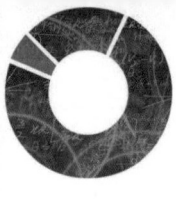
If you trust me, and take the seven steps of TSC, you can absolutely expect rapid weight loss, energy throughout the day, lots of lean muscle mass, lowered body-fat percentage, and physical well-being, including lowered blood glucose levels, lowered cholesterol, and risk of heart attack, stroke, and diabetes.

Your quality of life will improve tremendously, and you will feel a more vibrant spirituality, and a closer connection and presence within, as well as with Him and your relationships... With skyrocketing self confidence you may find yourself able to take on brand new challenges and adventures. Success is invigorating!

Or, if you'd rather, you can stay right where you're at, in your comfort zone. As the saying goes, if nothing changes, nothing changes. You can expect more of the same disappointing results, or worse.

You may experience obesity, chronic fatigue, sickness, diabetes, high cholesterol, anxiety, depression, and low self-esteem. You might spend tons of money on medications simply to mask the symptoms, with nothing ever getting to the root of the matter.

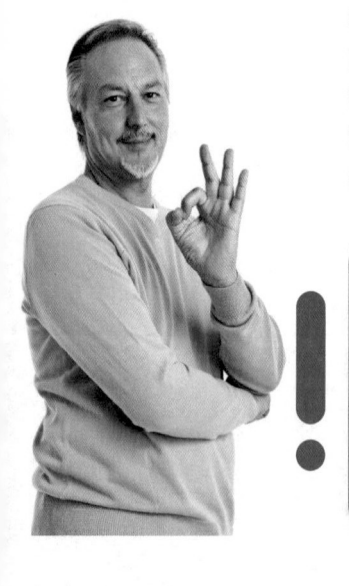

The choice is yours, but I hope you'll join me and take the first step in Chapter One by developing a *The Shepherd's Code* mindset. You'll learn just what *TSC* mindset will do for you and why it makes sense to give it a try.

 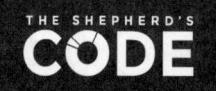

> *Though the mountains be shaken and the hills be removed, yet my unfailing love for you will not be shaken nor my covenant of peace removed.*
>
> **Isaiah 54:10**

Until you change the way you think about food, nothing else will matter.

Chapter One will help you do it by explaining how and why *TSC* can work for you, and why it makes sense to give it a try.

STEP 1: DEVELOP THE SHEPHERD'S CODE MINDSET

"I can't watch you kill yourself anymore, Krissie," my mother said. "Where did my beautiful daughter go? When you turn sideways, you disappear.

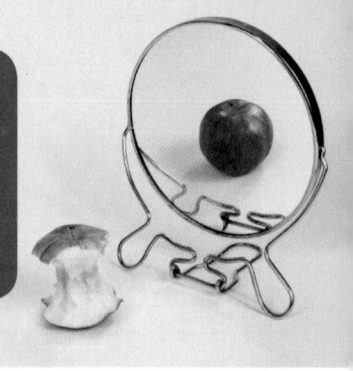

> You look gray. Your hair is awful. I love you so much, but if you don't go to rehab right now, I have to cut you off. We can't support you financially anymore, so you have a choice."

Wow, those words were quite the wake-up call.

Approximately 20 years ago, I was thin, but I wasn't healthy. I was what you call skinny-fat and basically dying. I had very serious eating disorders known as bulimia and anorexia. I was bingeing and purging up to six times a day. I hated to cook, so anything that was in a package or anything you could order in, I ordered, ate it, and threw it up. I spent so much money on binge food, only to vomit it up.

Before work, I'd drive to Burger King and order French toast sticks (4), pancakes (3) and 3 or 4 bacon, egg and cheese sandwiches!!! I'd hurry home to scarf down all the food, then quickly vomit it back up! Then, I'd be ready to go to work.

  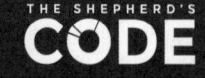

I remember thinking that I couldn't go on like that anymore, and that I'd die if I continued that behavior.

 It was scary and difficult, but I made the decision to go for 35 days of rehab in Orlando, Florida.

It was known as one of the best rehabs in the United States. I thought, "Okay, let's give this a shot. I have nothing to lose and everything to gain."

When I got there, it was interesting. I saw many overweight people. Not just overweight, but obese—300 or 400 pounds; those people had a food addiction too, but they didn't throw up. We all had an addiction; we just went about it in different ways, but food was the problem. We did all the groups together. We had individual therapy and group therapy.

They put everyone, regardless of weight, in the same category. So we ate breakfast, lunch, and dinner together. I distinctly remember being ravenous before each meal. It felt like I would just make it to mealtime without passing out. I kept thinking, "Is this how I'm going to have to live??" They removed sugar, wheat and flour from my diet, and this was good. However, I was starving because I wasn't consuming enough healthy fat. (Looking back, this is very clear.)

 Part of the program at rehab was to eliminate sugar, wheat, and flour from our food plans. I thought that was great because the sugary stuff was what I binged on all the time. However, I was an athlete, and I was starving, so my blood sugar was dropping too low, but nobody knew this at first.

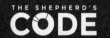

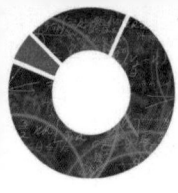
One day we went out on a pass to the movies, and in the middle of the movie, I started crying. My skin was clammy. I was sweaty. My friends said I looked really pale; I was shaky, and I thought, "What the heck is going on? Something is terribly wrong." They took me back to the center immediately, and the nurse tested my blood sugar. The number that came up was 37, which I found out is extremely low—borderline comatose, in fact.

The nurse gave me orange juice to raise my blood sugar quickly because fruit juice is loaded with sugar. Next, they altered my food plan. They added more fats to my regular breakfast, lunch and dinner. It was then that I realized I did need more fat and fewer carbs.

When I went home after discharge, I continued with the food plan, and I found a sponsor. I started going to meetings. They recommended 90 meetings in 90 days, so that's what I did.

Another amazing revelation that rehab introduced was a relationship with a 'higher power'. I was raised Catholic and believed in God but had no *relationship* with God. I really didn't 'know' Jesus. I knew some of the miracles he had performed and that he died on the cross and rose again but I didn't 'know' him.

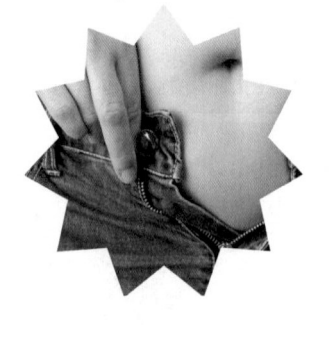

I asked myself how do you get to know someone? My answer was pretty simple. You talk to them, spend time with them and read about them. So, I began to talk to Jesus. Sometimes through prayer and sometimes just a conversation as if he was sitting right next to me. I began to read more of the New Testament. I studied Matthew, Mark, Luke

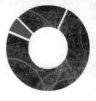

and John first. Then, I moved on to Acts, Romans, Corinthians, etc. The ironic thing that I noticed immediately was that Jesus encouraged eating fat! I was blown away. For example, in the story about the Prodigal Son, a fatted calf (the fattest) was used for the huge celebration to honor the son who found his way home.

This discovery was so exciting. I delved into the Old testament as well and discovered again that fat was recommended to us as food. In the whole Cain and Abel story, for example, God preferred Abel's gift of an animal over Caan's gift of grain. I felt even more sure that eating these "healing fats" was not only biblically sound but healing for my body.

"Foods with high fat content tend to taste amazing because many different flavors dissolve in fats. Butter especially works as an excellent carrier for a wide variety of flavors, including spices, vanilla and other fat soluble ingredients. The human body is also genetically programed to seek out high energy foods. Because of this, fatty foods are inherently perceived as more flavorful." (footnote, Boyers CHNC)

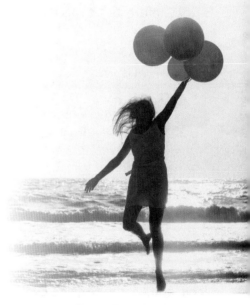

After about six months of no sugar, wheat, or flour, I noticed something. I noticed that when I ate potatoes, rice, corn, bananas, beans, or any kind of starchy substance, I didn't feel so well. I felt bloated and uncomfortable. I was listening to my body for the first time in my life!

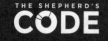

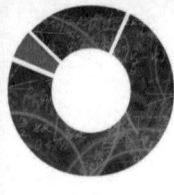
Due to the nature of my disease, "at times it (was) difficult to differentiate the truth from the false," as the AA Big Book says, but I had to trust what my body was telling me.

My roommate in rehab was a gal named Susanna from Australia. About a year after rehab, we met up in New York City. We made reservations to enjoy some time together at a fancy restaurant. I was pretty nervous about it because normally when I went out to eat, it was a disaster. (I would eat and then throw up.) But this time, it was fine. It was great. I was able to order a meal easily, one that contained a protein and a fat that I needed. It was awesome. I felt free finally from my eating disorder, probably for the first time. It was a major test, being in a restaurant of that nature, but it was easy, and I was finally really happy.

> *... And you will have joy in every good thing which the Lord your God has given to you ...*
>
> **Deuteronomy 26:11**

I was truly a living miracle. Today, I buy healthy, inexpensive, wholesome food, and I eat it. Nothing goes to waste, and while it's not necessary to be an expert chef on *TSC*, I now enjoy creating things in the kitchen all the time. I had been obsessed with being thin my whole life and thought that low-fat, low-sugar, sugar-free foods were the answer, but I was dead wrong. I needed "healing fats", and I learned to love them.

 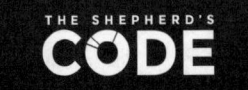

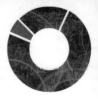

> *And take thou unto thee of all food that is eaten, and thou shalt gather it to thee; and it shall be for food for thee, and for them.*
>
> ***Genesis 6:21***

If I were to meet all those people I was in rehab with, I would tell them, "Guys, this is how you have to do it." My rehab was close to 20 years ago, and I am grateful for the experience and the wonderful people who worked there, but they missed the boat a little. It's kind of like giving an alcoholic one drink and saying, 'You'll be okay." No, not really. We can't have those unhealthy carbs in our system because even one creates a craving for more. When you remove carbs entirely and replace them with "healing fats", you feel so much better.

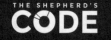

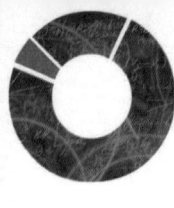

YOU ARE A MIRACLE WAITING TO HAPPEN

If you want to overcome whatever eating problem or disorder you have, if you want to feel better about yourself, if you want to develop a closer relationship with family, friends, and coworkers, and if you want to be fully present in your life to all the choices, to everything that is available to you, you need to start by changing your mindset. More specifically, you need to change the way you think about food and dieting by adopting a *TSC* mindset.

You don't have to starve. You don't have to feel deprived, and you certainly don't have to give up amazingly delicious food. You just need to believe that *TSC* can help you to get what you want. Listen to me, trust the process, and give it a chance to work.

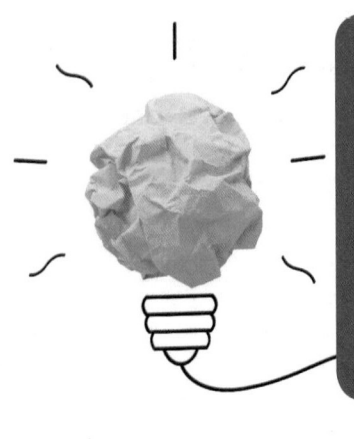

The Shepherd's Code System is the result of my many years of observation, experimentation, and experience. I changed my way of eating and that of the people I've worked with over the years, and by doing so I've arrived at a formula that works well for almost everyone.

You, my friend, are a miracle waiting to happen. The satisfaction and freedom that I now feel can be yours, too. I wrote this book for that purpose, and nothing would make me happier than for you to succeed with *TSC* as I, and so many others, already have.

 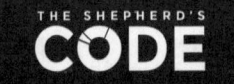

THE SHEPHERD'S CODE SYSTEM BASICS: TRUTH AND LIES ABOUT FOOD

The Shepherd's Code System includes using a lot of delicious "healing fats" and plenty of protein but no sugar, refined or processed foods, wheat, or flour. This makes *TSC* an extremely low-carb, moderate-protein, high-healing-fat lifestyle. The key to success with *TSC* is understanding and believing that (1) "healing fats" are good for you, (Omega 3's as opposed to Omega 6's) and (2) sugar (or glucose) from carbs (other than vitamin-rich vegetables) and excess protein are not.

What are "healing fats"? "Healing fats" are fats your body needs to operate at its peak level at all times, and you might be surprised to hear that the list of foods that contains them includes real bacon (not turkey bacon), real cream, real cheese, heavy whipping cream, and yes, real butter.

We've all been told, "Oh, don't eat too much butter; eat margarine, in-

 That's just ignorance or, in some cases, hype to keep us sick.

stead. Oh, don't eat bacon; eat turkey bacon."

TSC replaces carbs with "healing fats", and when you do that, your blood sugar stabilizes because you're not putting sugar into your system. And when you're eating lots of "healing fats" and moderate protein, you'll discover that fat is more satiating than any carb could ever be.

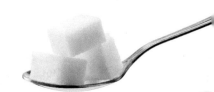

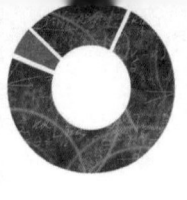

> *That same night they are to eat the meat roasted over the fire, along with bitter herbs,*
>
> **Exodus 12:8**

When you remove and replace carbs in your diet with "healing fats" found in meats, nuts, and certain oils, your body naturally uses those fats for energy instead of sugar (or glucose) from the carbs. That energy lasts longer because you have a much greater supply of fat than glucose in your body. The energy also remains more stable because your blood- sugar levels won't fluctuate as they would on a carbohydrate-based food plan. It's a really healthy, sound, and easy to eat diet that can be truly life changing.

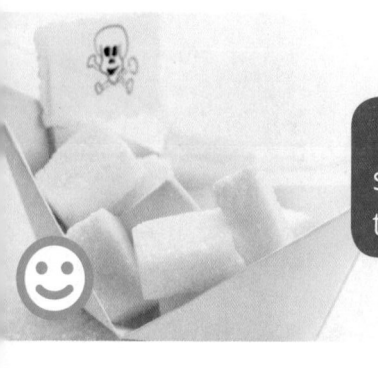

Wow! Isn't it crazy that we could be so easily brainwashed into believing that sugar is actually healthy?

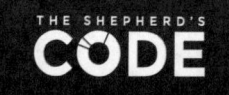

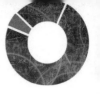

In 1944 President Roosevelt had a heart attack. His doctor blamed the president's diet. His doctor went on to vilify fat and was then influential in creating the American Standard Diet Food Pyramid (ASDFP).

As we know, the ASDFP tells us that fats should be the smallest portion on the pyramid and therefore what we should eat the least of! On the contrary, other evidence shows that carbs and sugar are the true villains concerning heart disease and other deadly conditions like diabetes.

The sugar industry has provided lots of money for researchers to simply "sugar coat" the truth!

According to newly released historical documents, during the 1960s, sugar industry leaders paid scientists great sums to play down the link between sugar and heart disease and to promote saturated fat as the culprit instead.

One major study has found that low-fat diets could actually raise the risk of early death by almost 25%. The Lancet study of 135,000 adults found those who cut back on fats had far shorter lives than those enjoying plenty of butter, cheese and meats.

There's no need for a deep, boring dive into the bowels of food science to explain the basics of *The Shepherd's Code System*, but you should know that foods are considered macro (or big) nutrients, and the big ones that we consume every day are protein, fat, and carbs.

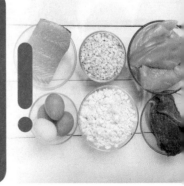

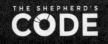

Protein comes from foods like meat, chicken, fish, and eggs. Fat is found in olive oil, which is kind of obvious, and avocados, nuts, and any kind of meat like bacon or other cuts that are very fatty. Of course, cream, real butter, cream cheese, or any kind of cheese are also good fat sources.

So, what about carbs? Carbohydrates are divided into simple carbs and complex carbs. The carbs that we enjoy on *TSC* are found in the vegetables like broccoli, green beans, cauliflower, and spinach—because anything green is great. The other kind of carbs like cookies, cake, pasta, and bread are not good. Those types of carbohydrates cause inflammation in the body, which can lead to a lot of complications.

Many diets advocate lots of protein and reduced carbs, and don't discuss much about fat consumption. There are some problems with these diets. First, eating so much protein can be a problem. For instance, have you heard that it's good to eat your body weight in grams of protein? Well, the average woman who weighs 140 or 150 pounds only needs around 70 grams of protein, which is only half of what would otherwise be recommended.

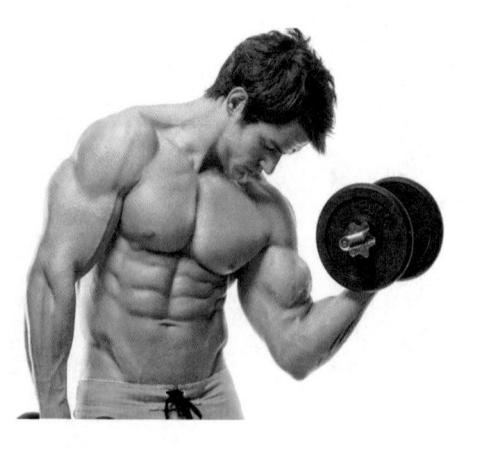

Unless you're trying to build a lot of muscle and compete in bodybuilding events (most people aren't), the average person simply needs half of their body weight in protein because too much protein is stored as sugar which is problematic.

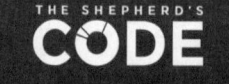

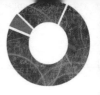

Bodybuilders who compete have a different mindset and goal for their diet. They're trying to achieve a specific look to win a competition. It's not necessarily healthy (they will tell you this themselves). I've competed before, and I got extremely sick on that diet. It taxes the body to the point of becoming weak and unwell, though you may look good.

> Remember, I was skinny, but I was unhealthy, so the diet that bodybuilders use is different from *TSC*, and they usually have someone called a prep person who helps them with it.

These nutrition experts know the ways a diet can reveal that very thin-skinned vascular look.

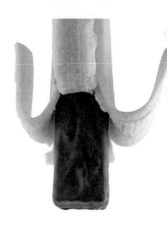

Most diets don't adequately explain carbohydrates. Many people think, "Oh, it's just bread; it's not a donut," or "It's just a banana," or "It's just a potato. What's wrong with that? If it's a vegetable or a fruit I can eat it. There's no sugar, right? It's not like it's candy." The truth is, those foods metabolize within the body as sugar. So, whether it's a potato, or a rice cake, or a banana, it all ends up the same as sugar.

It's the same thing across the board, whether it is protein or carbohydrates. Too much protein has the same end result of being stored as sugar. And any kind of starchy foods like bread, pasta, potatoes, rice, or quinoa all end up as sugar. Some foods, like quinoa, are hyped as super foods, but they are starches, just like rice, that turn into sugar in your body.

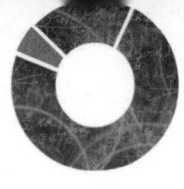
Sugar is a drug. That's the bottom line. Sugar is a drug, and you can become physically addicted to it. When I was in rehab, I started out in detox for three days. I had never done a drug—a street drug, or any other kind of drug—in my life. The drug that I was detoxing from was sugar.

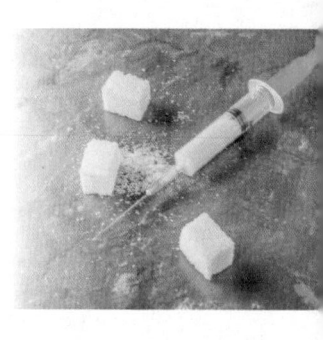

They put me in a different room from the regular rooms for three days and monitored me. I was constantly given lots of water and a sugar-free Gatorade. Gatorade, the kind that doesn't have sugar, helped keep my electrolytes up because withdrawing from sugar was extremely uncomfortable.

When they first put me along with my roommate in the detox room, I thought, "What is this?" They told me, "Honey, you have an addiction. Your addiction is to sugar." I thought, "No, I don't. I don't need to be in detox. I'm fine." They told me, "Just wait until tomorrow." I said, "Okay." They were anticipating a possible severe reaction because they eliminated the sugar, wheat, and flour that I was used to consuming every day.

"When we eat carbs, the body breaks them down into glucose (sugar). Fiber is the only carb that does NOT convert to glucose. When there is too much glucose floating around in the blood stream, lots of insulin gets released. This can lead to insulin resistance and make weight loss virtually impossible, no matter how hard we try!" (footnote, see Boyers CNHC)

I increased my intake of olive oil, avocados, cheese and nuts — all the good "healing fats". I had to eat double the amount of good fats at the

> While they decreased my sugar intake, they increased my fats, which balanced my sugar levels. Once they did that, I never had a drop again.

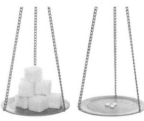

rehab because I was young, I was in my 20s, and I was an athlete. My natural metabolism was through the roof. Because I was listening to my body for the first time and not to the misinformed doctors, I knew to increase my fat intake.

We don't need sugar in our diets. When we were hunters and gatherers, we didn't have many sources of sugar. The sweetest thing we had in those days was fruit—like a fig or a berry, and berries are fine to eat on *TSC*. They're the fruit that we recommend. They're also great antioxidants.

The fats we need do the important work of leveling our blood sugar. When your blood sugar is level, you are satiated; you're not starving, and you can maintain for an extended period of time.

It takes much longer to break down fat than it does to break down a simple or complex carbohydrate. So, besides consuming a lot more "healing fats", you need to eliminate bad carbs: pasta, bread, cake, cereal, oatmeal, and anything that is considered a starch.

Protein is excellent for you in moderate amounts, but don't go crazy and eat so much that your body converts the excess amount into sugar. The only *TSC System*-approved carbs are vegetables. Our bodies need them to function properly, and they don't break down into sugar like other carbs do.

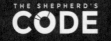

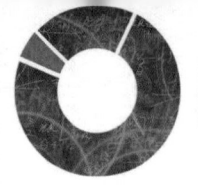
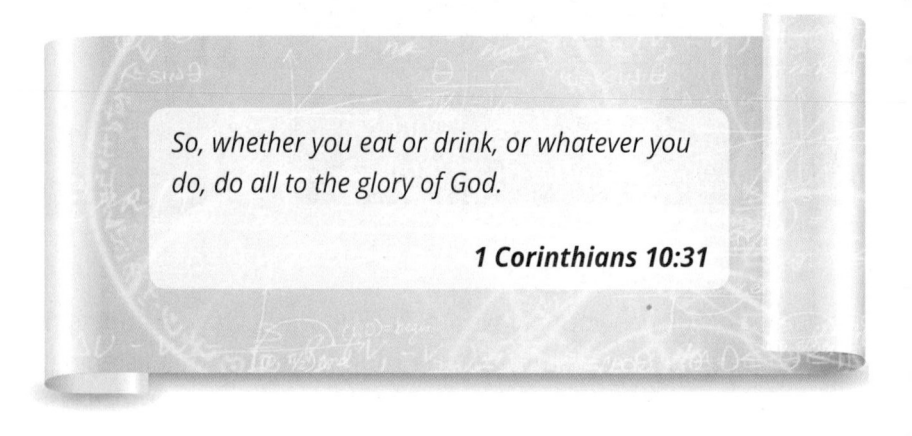

So, whether you eat or drink, or whatever you do, do all to the glory of God.

1 Corinthians 10:31

BENEFITS OF THE SHEPHERD'S CODE SYSTEM

There are too many benefits of *TSC System* to list, especially when spiritual and emotional ones are considered (as they should be), but some of the biggest and most obvious benefits of embracing *TSC* are as follows:

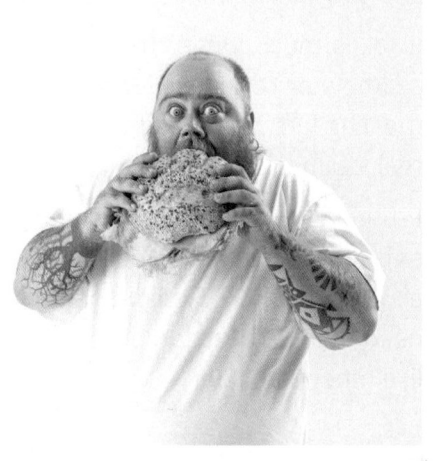

The first benefit is natural appetite suppression. When I began eating a high fat, moderate protein, low carb diet, I was no longer hungry. I could go 8 to 10 hours without food and felt great. I never even realized when I forgot to eat because I was so satiated!

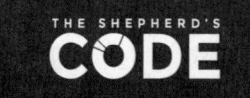

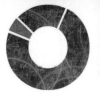

This lifestyle works better than any pill for appetite control. The "healing fats" are so satiating, you do not feel hunger. When you do feel hungry, listen to your body and eat. For years, I searched for the perfect pill to curb my appetite and get rid of my craving for sugar. This lifestyle was the answer.

> *The afflicted shall eat and be satisfied; those who seek him shall praise the Lord! May your hearts live forever!*
>
> **Psalm 22:26**

The second benefit is the opportunity for spontaneous fasting. Who would have thought fasting could be easy? Because your blood sugar is level and stable, you can go many hours without food. Water is essential, of course, but food is not. I can do a 12/8, 16/8 intermittent fast and sometimes a 24/8! Fasting cleanses the body and adds to your mental clarity.

It allows your body to hit those fat stores for energy so that the fat melts off your body! When I had tried to fast in the past, it was very difficult. I'd feel light headed, dizzy, nauseous and weak. When fasting with this lifestyle, I felt just the opposite. We have 90% more fat to use for energy than glucose. That's a large energy source!!

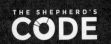

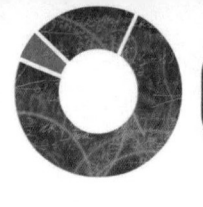
That your fasting may not be seen by others but by your Father who is in secret. And your Father who sees in secret will reward you.

Matthew 6:18

Here's a quick story about one of my attempts to starve the fat off me when I was in my twenties. I was working as a social worker for the state, and my salary was pitiful. So, I took a part time modeling job for a local boutique. I signed on with a modeling agency and would get weekend opportunities like fashion shows and print work. I was paranoid about gaining weight and not fitting into the sizes I had to wear. I decided to fast. Well, it did not go well! I was eating one Fig Newton every other day!! A Fig Newton is filled with sugar and carbs!!! Anyway, I got to the job and ran back stage to change. I was so starved and weak, I had no idea what was going on. The gal backstage showed me my five outfits and told me to hurry because I was up in two minutes!! I quickly threw on what I thought was the outfit to model. I ended up wearing red leggings with a striped jacket and thought, "This looks ridiculous, but ok." As I headed out to the stage to do my 'walk,' the woman backstage grabbed my arm and said,"Honey, what on earth are you wearing? That is not the correct ensemble!! You look ridiculous!"

There you have it, I was so light headed, dizzy and starved, I could not even put on clothing that matched!!!! When I fast the right way with nutritional ketosis, I have abounding mental acuity and zero brain fog!!!

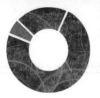

The third benefit of *TSC* is mental clarity. We have 39% greater blood flow as fat burners than those who are sugar burners (using glucose for fuel). When the brain utilizes ketones for energy from the body burning fat for fuel, mental clarity and sharpness greatly improves. You feel amazing! There is no other way to describe it! Feeling alert and sharp even through that 3 pm lull in the day is fantastic. It adds up to better performance at work and a better presence for my family and friends.

The fourth unexpected benefit is sound sleep. How many nights have you tossed and turned, unable to fall asleep? I bet you have tried prescription medicine, melatonin and counting sheep! I too have tried it all. Not until I began eating a high-fat, low-carb diet did I actually have a good, full night's sleep. When your blood sugar is stabilized, it's easier to sleep. There are no cravings or crazy hunger pangs keeping you awake. Your body is content and doing what it needs to do naturally, sleep.

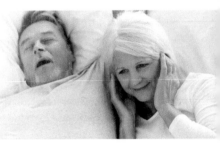

I lay down and slept; I woke again, for the Lord sustained me.

Psalm 3:5

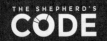

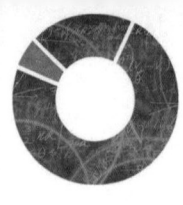
A fifth benefit, referenced earlier, is blood sugar stabilization. I was diagnosed with hypoglycemia in my twenties. Hypoglycemia occurs when there is low blood-sugar. Hyperglycemia is the opposite. It is an overabundance of sugar in the blood. Anyway, I had to eat every two hours or I would faint. Little did I know it was because I was avoiding fat like the plague and consuming only refined, processed foods!!!

Eating sugar makes you want sugar. The cravings are off the charts. You never feel satisfied and are always left "wanting more." For example, I would eat a bowl of Cheerios and milk with sliced apple for breakfast. Doesn't sound too bad, right??? Wrong!! Cheerios are terrible for you! Everything is filled with sugar in that breakfast. Even the apple with naturally occurring fructose was not a wise choice. I'd be starving an hour after I ate.

Today, I enjoy breakfast and can have a Keto Bagel or bacon and eggs or avocado and celery. These choices are very wise! The high fat and protein keep my blood glucose levels stable. I don't get hungry for at least 5 to 6 hours after I eat breakfast.

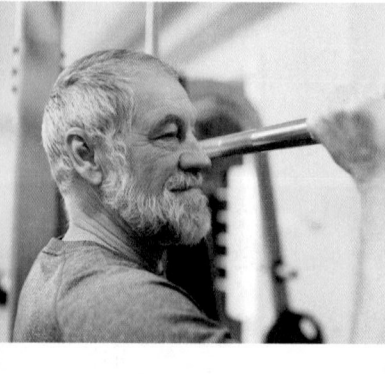

The sixth unexpected benefit is an increase in strength. I could lift a good 25 lbs or more on almost any exercise. My deadlift rose from 163 lbs. to a whopping 200 lbs.!! I only weighed 125 lbs. at the time so this was impressive as heck! When our muscles are fueled with "healing fats", they work better. Sugar, grains and carbs can give us a burst of energy but nothing sustainable. When eating a diet of high fat, endurance is long lasting and easily sustainable.

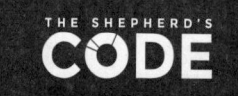

The seventh unexpected benefit is greatly reduced inflammation throughout the body. The C-Reactive Protein (CRP) is what indicates inflammation. It needs to be around 1.0 for optimal health. If you do not know what your CRP level is, you might want to get it checked out soon! Inflammation will wreak havoc on the body in the form arthritis, GI issues, headaches and autoimmune diseases. If your CRP level is greater than 1.0, you should consider a high-fat, moderate-protein, low-carb lifestyle.

The eighth unexpected benefit is abounding energy! My energy is literally through the roof! I rise at 5:00 am every morning and stretch, drink my water with lemon, get the coffee going, empty the dishwasher, get my son up for school, feed him and take him to school all before 7:30am!! Thank goodness I have the energy from this lifestyle to sustain me throughout the day!

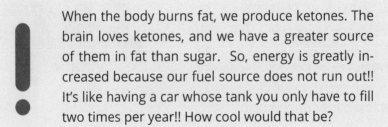

When the body burns fat, we produce ketones. The brain loves ketones, and we have a greater source of them in fat than sugar. So, energy is greatly increased because our fuel source does not run out!! It's like having a car whose tank you only have to fill two times per year!! How cool would that be?

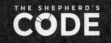

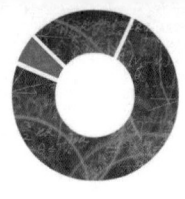

The ninth unexpected benefit is the elimination of LDL particles. You might be thinking, "What the heck are LDLs?? Well it's the size of the LDL particles that matter, not the number. LDLs come in two forms: light and fluffy or small and dense. Ask your doctor for the test that shows the size of the particles, it's much more significant to your overall health. The small and dense particles easily penetrate and can be considered more dangerous for a cardiovascular event. Your numbers (of the small dense LDLs) should decrease greatly the longer you stay on the high-fat low-carb lifestyle.

Finally, the tenth unexpected benefit is the resolution of skin issues. I had a client named MacKenzie. She was a young gal in her early twenties. Her acne was a source of pain and embarrassment. It really affected her self-esteem. After just one month on the high-fat, low-carb plan, her skin looked amazing! She was so happy! Also, issues like cystic acne, dry skin and even wrinkles look better and feel better on this plan.

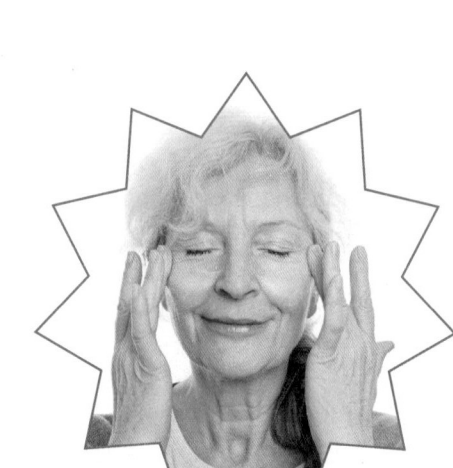

A bonus benefit for some is improved fertility. Studies of women on high-fat, low-carb, moderate-protein diets like *The Shepherd's Code System* were able to conceive much more quickly than those who weren't.

Fortunately, the truth about "healing fats" and *TSC* is starting to reveal itself because it's becoming too hard to deny. In a recent groundbreaking study by the American Journal of Clinical Nutrition, researchers discovered that "healing fats"–or what they called "healthy fats"–are good for you. More specifically, the study found that middle-aged men who ate low levels of carbohydrates and high levels of saturated fats lost weight.

The diet also lowered their blood pressure and glucose levels, leading them to conclude that, contrary to popular belief, high-fat, low-carb diets like *TSC System* can not only make people look and feel better, they can help prevent diabetes, heart risk, and other debilitating conditions and diseases.

Considering the study's findings and the weight of other evidence pointing in a similar direction, Professor Sharif Sultan, a heart specialist from the University of Ireland, stated:

"We urgently need to overturn current dietary guidelines. People should not be eating high carbohydrate diets as they have been told over the past decade. Instead, our diets should be largely based on good quality, high-fat foods. This will prevent the rising epidemic of type 2 diabetes and reverse the growing numbers of people suffering weight-related heart problems."

He further opined, quite accurately, that diets high in carbohydrates and sugars are the primary driver of the obesity epidemic. There will, no doubt, be more studies like this to come. I hope this book serves to further bring the truth to light as well.

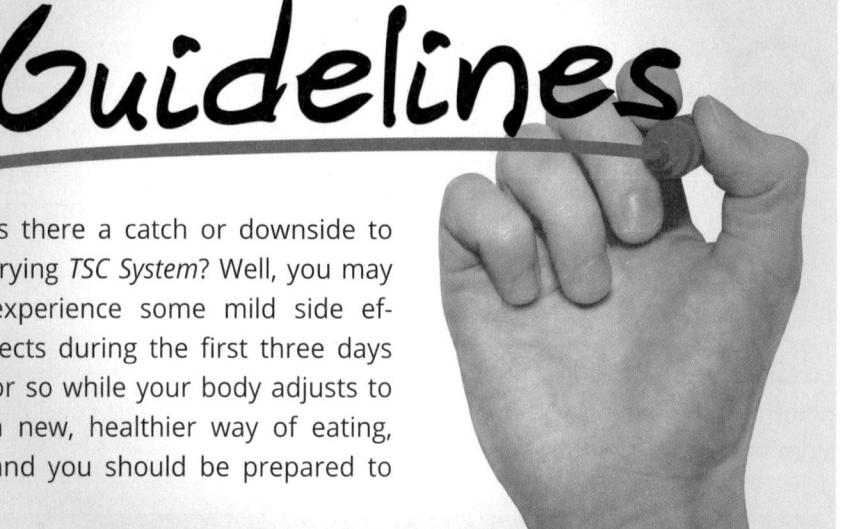

Guidelines

Is there a catch or downside to trying *TSC System*? Well, you may experience some mild side effects during the first three days or so while your body adjusts to a new, healthier way of eating, and you should be prepared to be a little uncomfortable at the start. These discomforts may include fatigue, irritability, and/or constipation. (Tip: Take some magnesium to bounce back more quickly.) And if you're a real carb lover, your transition may be slightly more challenging than someone who doesn't eat many carbs before they begin *TSC*. But don't let some minor temporary side effects discourage you! Power through the first few days and enjoy these amazing benefits!

 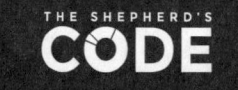

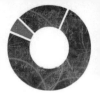

WHAT TO EAT

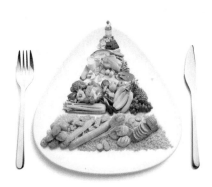

If you adopt a *TSC* mindset and try this food plan, you will get to eat the most amazing foods. How do grilled hamburgers with lots and lots of extra cheese and bacon sound to you? Just drop the carb-filled bun and go to town. Another example of food you get to eat is dark chocolate—85% cocoa or higher is wonderful!

You can have real cream. You can get your strawberries out, squirt the real cream all over them, and go to town. You can eat these wonderful foods and "healing fats" guilt-free on *The Shepherd's Code System* if you eliminate the bad carbs. It's a tradeoff, but a good one!

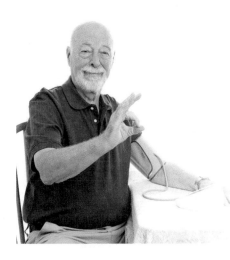

Other super-low-carb, healing-fat and/or moderate-protein foods to eat and enjoy on *TSC* include natural fats like real butter and olive oil, eggs, bacon, meat, fish and seafood, nuts, vegetables, and chicken. All you have to do to become a fat-melting machine is eat this kind of food and avoid the bad carbs.

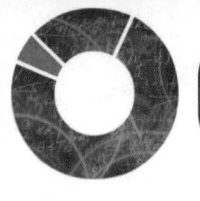

To be fair, some foods and drinks are tricky to categorize (in part, due to media manipulation and corporate shenanigans) and lead to innocent mistakes, which is why I'm going to give you a heads-up on some of them now.

Fruit is loaded with carbs, for example—it's nature's candy—and fruit juice is even worse. Avoid them, especially bananas and grapes. So are those cafe lattes and cappuccinos at Starbucks, or any other coffee with all that milk and sugar; go with black coffee (with a little whipped cream on top if you like), instead. Lots of water is highly recommended on *TSC*, but not the kind of water with added sugar, and there's a lot of it out there. And, while most nuts are a tremendous source of "healing fats" and relatively low in carbs, avoid carb-heavy cashews completely.

What about snacks like crackers that seem to throw so many people off their diet, whatever it is? You know how it is–once you eat one cracker, you want another and another until the bag is empty. You never get full or completely satiated.

That doesn't need to happen if you choose a "healing fat" snack, instead. After you eat a handful of macadamia nuts or almonds with salt, for example, you become satiated, and you don't want to eat any more. There's no craving because the fat in those nuts is satiating. That doesn't happen with crackers, cakes, and cookies in the same way, does it?

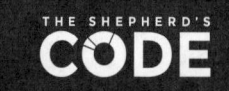

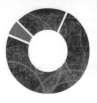

Other *TSC System* approved snacks to consider include cold cuts (black forest ham, sliced turkey and sliced roast beef), cheese or cheese sticks (with no bread), real whipped cream, avocado, olives, and eggs.

> Then there's the other major stumbling block for many people trying to follow TSC: Alcohol.

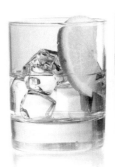
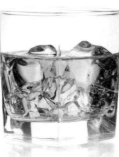
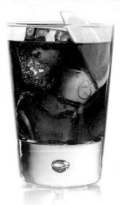

I'll cover this in more detail in Chapter 5 (about resisting temptations), but for now, the best advice I can give you is to (a) abstain from drinking altogether, (b) opt for zero-carb alcohol like vodka, whisky, tequila or rum, either without a mixer or with soda water, not fruit juice or something like that; or (c) drink anything else in moderation—less is more.

You can disregard my guidance about developing a *TSC* mindset and stop here at Step 1, but don't expect anything other than what you're experiencing now—like being overweight, being chronically tired, intensely fatigued, irritable, and sleep deprived—at least not in the long-term.

Maybe you have sinus issues, asthma, or chronic pain, too. Well, I hate to say it, but those things are highly likely to continue plaguing you if you aren't willing to get out of your comfort zone and try something new.

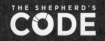

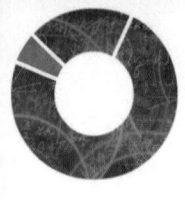

Other food plans or diets like Jenny Craig, Nutrisystem, or Slimgenics may help you lose weight for a while, but here's the ugly truth: You're likely to eventually put the pounds back on because you haven't really learned or changed anything. You're just restricting your calories and slowing your metabolism. When you begin to integrate eating regular food again (and at some point, you must), the weight will come back, and usually even more weight comes with it.

With *TSC System*, you can expect lasting, permanent results. It's a life-style, not a diet.

So, what are you waiting for?

Maybe you're worried about whether you can really stop eating carbs for any extended period because you love sug-ary foods and always end up giving in to your cravings. Well, don't worry. Just take Step Two of *The Shepherd's Code System* and free yourself from your sugar addiction, as I and so many others have. Chapter Two will show you how to do it more quickly and easily than you ever thought possible, with a little help from "healing fats".

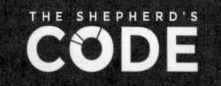

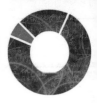

STEP 2: FREE YOURSELF FROM FOOD ADDICTION

Before I discovered *TSC*, I was working as a law enforcement officer in the city of Camden, New Jersey. Camden is one of the three worst cities in the country for drugs, crime and murder. Most of the population is in their 20's.

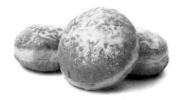

We often had meetings on the latest laws, regulations and codes. During these meetings, there was always some kind of sugary food to share, usually donuts. They were dripping in chocolate with sugar and cream and jelly. The white powdery sugar looked so tantalizing in the middle of the table as I sat there in a trance-like state dreaming of donuts!!

All I could focus on was the donuts. I could not take my eyes off them. I kept imagining eating them and then running to the bathroom to re-gurgitate. Those donuts made it difficult to focus on what my boss was saying or what the officers were saying during these meetings. I secretly wished I was alone with my delicious treats. Since I was bulimic at the time, my heart would pound heavily in my chest. My mouth watered as cold sweat covered me while I pictured myself eating them all and then, of course, getting rid of them in the bathroom.

 "Every 62 minutes one person dies as a direct result of an eating disorder."

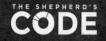

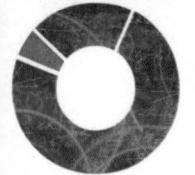
According to the Public Library of Science (PLOS) Journal, a peer-reviewed open access journal, a study about rats stated that when the rats were given a choice between cocaine and sugar, the rats chose sugar. They chose the sugar 94% of the time over the cocaine. The findings concluded that the attraction to intense sweetness can surpass attraction to cocaine. This demonstrates clearly the insidious craving that sugar produces.

When I was in my 20's, I had to go to rehab to overcome my own addiction to food. I had no idea how to eat. I had no choice but to go because I didn't know what to eat or how to fix healthy food. The staff at the rehab fed me the food, or it was right there, and I didn't have to think about it or cook it. I needed this extreme situation for change to happen.

Rehab was hard!

I had no idea how to feed myself. We ate at the same times every day, and those of us with food issues ate in a different part of the cafeteria than those with drug/alcohol issues. We were taught how to weigh and measure our food. Back then, this was used as a tool for not putting too much or too little on our plates.

I found myself starving before each meal. Remember, I was in my 20s and an athlete and had a metabolism of a racehorse! No one considered this when putting me on the same food plan as everyone else present! When my blood sugar plummeted one day out on a pass, the clinicians took notice! They upped my fat intake immediately! It helped, and the rest of my stay was much easier.

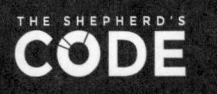

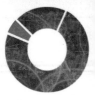

 This experience represented the beginning of my journey in discovering how to really eat. I learned how to nourish the body, fuel the body, and feed the body.

It was the beginning of finding a lasting and permanent solution to my eating disorder and freeing myself from an addiction to unhealthy food.

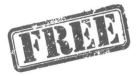

Eventually, after years of trial and error and turning to my nutritional journals for inspiration, my journey led me to discover *TSC System*, and it was truly a miracle.

After just three days of eating the food on *TSC*, my blood sugar was much more stable. I didn't even think about food, and I could really be present for my life.

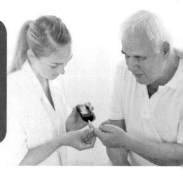

If I had known about *TSC* prior to going to rehab, I would have tried it and possibly avoided rehab altogether. I would have done everything that it recommended. I would have bought the food that it said to purchase and followed the sample meals. I believe I would not have had to go to an extreme environment like rehab if I had known this diet existed.

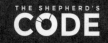

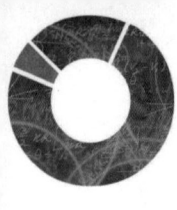
HOW ADDICTED TO UNHEALTHY FOOD ARE YOU?

If you're like me, you don't want your days consumed with food or to be constantly thinking about or obsessed with food. What am I going to eat? What am I not going to eat? It's the same issue all the time.

You want to be free from addiction to food of any kind because you want to be in control of your own life, diet, and decision-making. Any person who is addicted to sugar understands the pain and anguish of not being able to satisfy that sugar craving immediately due to work situations or events with kids, and so on. It's sheer torture.

Do not love the world or the things in the world. If anyone loves the world, the love of the Father is not in him. For all that is in the world—the desires of the flesh and the desires of the eyes and pride in possessions—is not from the Father but is from the world. And the world is passing away along with its desires, but whoever does the will of God abides forever.

1 John 2:15-17

COMMONALITIES BETWEEN ADDICTION TO SUGAR AND OTHER DRUGS

First,

both sweet tastes and cocaine stimulate dopamine, the feel-good chemical found naturally in our brains.

Second,

cross-dependence on sugar and drugs has been observed.

Third,

neuroimaging found that the brain of obese individuals addicted to sweets mimicked exactly the images of those addicted to drugs of abuse, like cocaine, for example (see notes).

 Wow, no wonder I was put into a detox unit!

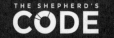

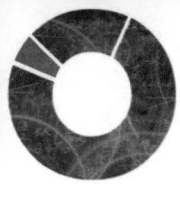

HOW TO SET YOURSELF FREE

You can free yourself from food addiction and the obsession of food by reading *TSC System* and simply following the steps and food recommendations.

> *Thou shall not eat too much honey.*
>
> **Proverbs 25:16**

You are the only person who can decide whether you need to go to a structured, safe environment to learn how to eat or if you might succeed by following *TSC System*. If you choose to follow the book, you will want to remove all the trigger foods—all the sugar, all the donuts, all the processed foods, all the stuff that you binge on or you like to eat compulsively. Get it out of the house!

> *The truth shall set you free.*
>
> **John 8:32**

CLEAN OUT THE KITCHEN

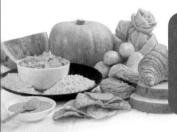

Remove all the trigger foods like bread, pasta, sugar, cereal, cookies, cake and candy. If it's in a packet, sack it. When in doubt, throw it out.

It's so important to stop eating these foods completely—cold turkey—because they are your drug. If you were a recovering alcoholic or addict, you would not continue to have alcohol or drugs in your home. The same applies to your trigger foods. You need to stop eating all foods that are carbs, the trigger foods. The sugary stuff, the pasta, the bread. It must stop completely. I was able to do this when I came to believe that a power greater than myself, God, could restore me to sanity. (AA Step)

Sugar of any kind fuels the food addiction. It creates a phenomenon of craving, and it puts you in a state of constant turmoil, internally and externally. You become a walking mess!

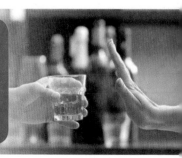

If you are an alcoholic trying to overcome an addiction to alcohol, you can't have the occasional shot and a beer. You must get it out of the house and try to avoid it elsewhere.

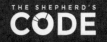

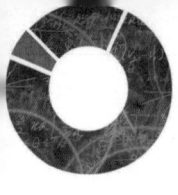
Several years ago, I met a lovely gal named Amy. When I met Amy, she was addicted to alcohol and overweight. Amy was only 24 years old and a full-blown alcoholic. I was her trainer and soon became her friend and confidante.

I was extremely concerned for Amy's health and well-being. She would come to the gym, reeking of alcohol. I was scared she might pass out or have a heart attack if I pushed her too hard physically! I would gently suggest time and time again the idea of going to AA, a detox unit, rehab, and/or counseling. At the time, Amy was not ready.

One day Amy's mother called me and told me Amy was withdrawing from alcohol at home. Her mom explained it was painful to watch. Amy would vomit, shake, sweat profusely and cry hour after hour. Thank God, after four days, she was out of the woods. Amy began attending meetings, got a sponsor and admitted to me and her mom the exact nature of her problem. She was well on her way to living a clean and sober lifestyle. I was so happy and grateful for Amy's courage and strength to let go of her addiction to booze.

Today, Amy has almost three years in recovery. She looks beautiful and still trains with me three times per week. Although Amy is free from her addiction to alcohol, she is in chains with something else! Amy is addicted to food, sugary sweets, in particular. I've watched her work so hard in the gym only to blow it on Reese's Peanut Butter Cups when she gets home. She has starved herself, decreased calories, stopped eating by 6pm in the evening, and tried energy drinks with loads of caffeine, all in an effort to lose weight. None of these futile tactics had worked.

I finally decided to ask Amy if she would try *The Shepherd's Code System*.

 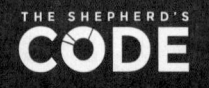

She was skeptical at first because it meant she could eat butter, cream and dark chocolate!! How could this possibly work for me she asked?? I explained that she would be decreasing carbs in her food plan to 20g or less every day. I explained to her the process of turning her body into a fat-burning machine instead of a sugar-burning machine. I also gave her a shopping list of foods to buy and a sample of what one day looks like on *TSC System*. She was thrilled!

Amy was so enthusiastic about *TSC* that she started right away. As a result of Amy's brave efforts, she is losing weight the right way for the first time in her life! Amy explained that she had tried Slimgenics years ago and lost weight. However, she gained it all back because she had no idea how to eat!

With *TSC System*, you learn how to eat real food. Nothing is prepackaged or processed. You eat wholesome real food every day! The excitement on Amy's face has been all the thanks I've needed. This young woman has taken control of her life and can now help others do the same.

> *Do not neglect to do good and to share what you have, for such sacrifices are pleasing to God.*
>
> **Hebrews 13:16**

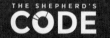

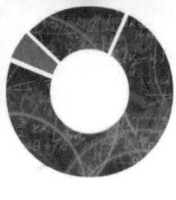

BRAD'S STORY

Another client who freed himself from food addiction using *TSC System* was named Brad. Brad was a 46-year-old father of five who went through a very ugly divorce and turned to food for comfort. Sweets became the best friend that he would turn to during stressful times.

When he first came to me, Brad weighed in at 195 lbs with 19% body fat. At 5'8", this was not a healthy weight. Brad admitted that he felt bone tired, fatigued and out of breath when he would walk up his stairs.

One day, he was walking in the mall and passed a mirror. He was stunned by what he saw in his reflection. The first thing he noticed was a big, protruding belly. He couldn't believe he was looking at himself. He went home, stripped down to his underwear and stared into his mirror. He thought, "Something has got to be done!" He had always been a lean, fit guy. He talked to some of his male and female friends who had lost weight successfully and asked, "How did you do it?" They replied, "We cut carbs!" He decided to remove carbs as in, bread, pasta, rice, potatoes, bananas etc....

He also began going to the gym four to five times per week for 30-minute sessions each time.

Brad hired me as his personal trainer to help him meet his goals. He took a picture of himself in his underwear and stuck it to the door of his refrigerator. Every time he felt hungry, depressed or bored, he would look at the picture on the door of his refrigerator and make a better choice. Instead of turning to empty calories, he did something good for himself; he drank two full glasses of water.

> *But whoever drinks of the water that I will give him will never be thirsty again. The water that I will give him will become in him spring of water welling up to eternal life.*
>
> ***John 4:14***

The picture was an extremely helpful deterrent. After four months, he had increased his muscle mass, and his body fat percentage dropped to 11%. His friends and family all commented on how slim and fit he looked. People started asking him, "What are you doing?" **He replied, "I decreased the carbs in my diet and increased the good fat.**

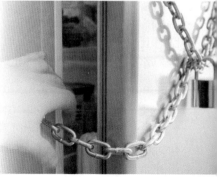

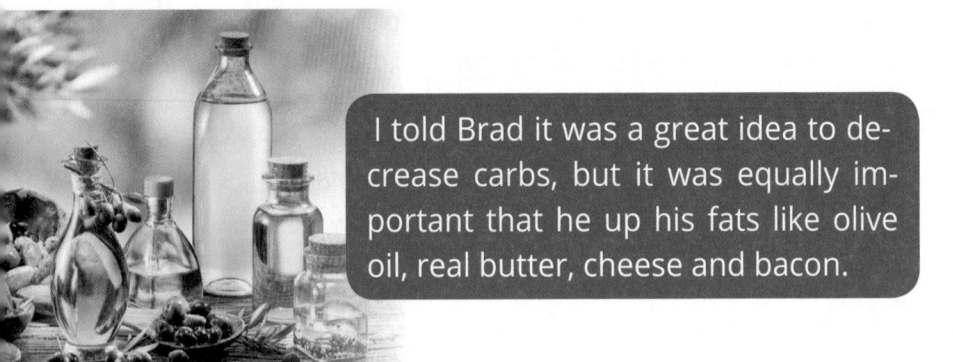

> I told Brad it was a great idea to decrease carbs, but it was equally important that he up his fats like olive oil, real butter, cheese and bacon.

When Brad embraced "healing fats", he said he never felt better in his life! He told me he had increased energy, no fatigue and was never out of breath when running up the stairs anymore! He also claimed to have great mental clarity. This is important to mention because at age 14, Brad's best friend accidentally shot him in the head. The two teenage boys were looking at the gun with wonder and awe. Even though both boys were excellent gunmen, their zeal and excitement caused them to be careless.

When Brad's friend was handing him the gun to admire, the gun fired. The doctors told Brad he would never walk or talk again. He proved them wrong. I mention these details because *TSC* helps with brain function. Brad said it was amazing how clearly he can think and not be bothered by "fuzzy" thinking or "brain fog" anymore. Today Brad is a strapping 166 lbs. with a mere 9% body fat. He has adopted *TSC* as a lifestyle!

You may experience some symptoms of fatigue and some irritability, but hang in there and don't surrender to cravings or comfort food because your reward is coming soon! The more time and space you put between consuming sugar/carbs, the more your craving for those foods will diminish.

 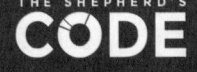

> When you begin *The Shepherd's Code System*, you may be a little uncomfortable for the first three days, especially if you're a person who loves unhealthy carbs, has a bagel for breakfast, a sandwich for lunch, and pasta for dinner.

By day four on *TSC*, your discomfort will dissipate or disappear completely, your food addiction will fade away, and you'll begin to feel amazingly well. In fact, you may feel better than you've ever felt in your life because you'll be at or near a state of "ketosis," which you must experience to truly understand.

Ketosis is simply a metabolic state where your body burns fat instead of sugar (glucose) for energy. This happens when you drop your carbohydrate intake to 20g or less and increase your "healing fats" intake dramatically. Your food plan will look like this: 75% "healing fat", 20% protein and 5% carbs.

REPLACE CARBS WITH HEALTHY FOOD AND "HEALING FATS"

I'm sure you don't like the idea of throwing away all those tasty, unhealthy foods and being a little uncomfortable for the first three days, but here's the good news: by day four you'll feel great and second, you'll be able to replace all that bad food with some of the most delicious "healing fats" you've ever tasted. These fats include hamburgers (not 97/3), bacon (real bacon), eggs, nuts, omelets with tons of cheese, butter, cream and a whole lot more. You can even put cheese on all your vegetables. How cool is that?

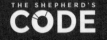

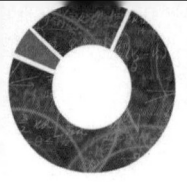
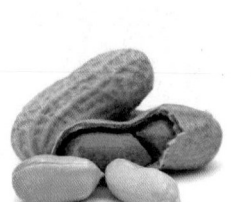

A healthy snack such as nuts (macadamia or almonds are best for *TSC*) not only satisfies hunger but improves health and longevity! Cardiologists have discovered that by consuming nuts, you are preparing your body to fight off diseases such as obesity, heart disease and even cancer.

The risk of respiratory diseases and diabetes can be cut in half by simply consuming an ounce of nuts.

Dagfinn Aune, of the School of Public Health at Imperial College, London, said, "We found a consistent reduction in risk across many different diseases, which is a strong indication there is a real underlying relationship between nut consumption and different health outcomes."

"It's quite a substantial effect for such a small amount of food." Nuts are considered a superfood because they possess anti-inflammatory qualities and are also high in protein and fiber. In research published in the journal of BMC Medicine Today, experts from Imperial and the Norwegian University of Science and Technology found eating them was associated with a reduction in disease risk.

Mr. Aune said: "In nutritional studies so far much of the research has been on the big killers such as heart disease, stroke and cancer, but now we're starting to see data for other diseases."

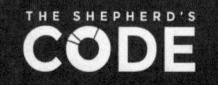

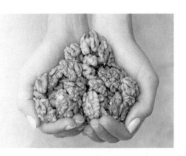

Eating a handful of nuts per day can aid in weight loss because they satiate hunger and cravings.

According to Cardiologist Dr. Aseem Malhotra, "This analysis adds further value to scores of clinical studies that reveal the positive health impact of regular nut consumption. Their mechanism of benefit appears to be through anti-inflammatory properties. It's time doctors started prescribing nuts to patients which will not only help prevent heart attacks and deaths within a short space of time but combined with other lifestyle interventions would save the NHS billions."

Remember, a peanut is NOT a nut. Peanuts are legumes and can cause inflammation.

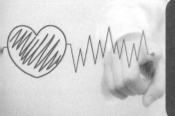

According to the Centers for Disease Control and Prevention, (see graph below) inactivity and obesity are the top two reasons for heart disease in America.

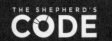

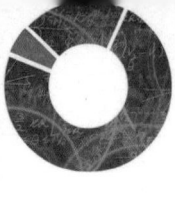
The Faces of Cardioascular Disease in America

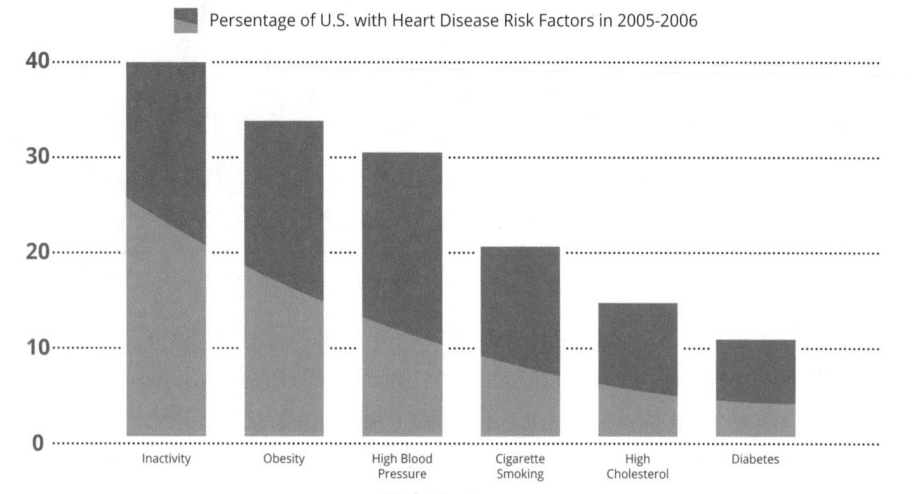

Persentage of U.S. with Heart Disease Risk Factors in 2005-2006

Risk Factors

(Bar chart values, left to right: Inactivity ~40, Obesity ~34, High Blood Pressure ~31, Cigarette Smoking ~21, High Cholesterol ~15, Diabetes ~11; y-axis marked 0, 10, 20, 30, 40)

FOLLOW THE FOOD PLAN

Once you've trashed the bad food and replaced it with tasty "healing fats", it's time to follow *TSC System's* recommended food plan and really crush it.

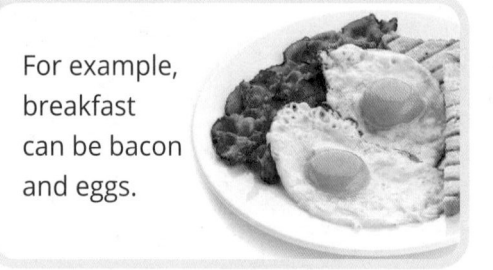

For example, breakfast can be bacon and eggs.

For a snack, you can have cheese sticks and almonds. Lunch can be tuna salad with lots of olive oil, salt, pepper. Another snack? An avocado with salt and pepper.

 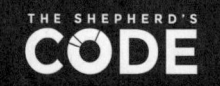

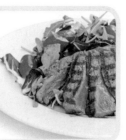

Dinner can be a steak and salad, and a snack in the evening could be full-fat yogurt and almond butter, mixed together. Delicious! There are so many options on *TSC*.

Once you have your food plan mapped out, you just need to go to the store, buy the food and begin. Absolutely never, ever feed yourself those trigger carbs that you ate prior to taking on *The Shepherd's Code System*.

You can continue to eat chicken, steak, fish, eggs, and pork. You may continue to eat any protein in moderation. You may be thinking, I thought protein was so great for the body? Yes, you are correct. Protein helps build muscle in our body. However, too much protein is stored as sugar! It's important to keep your protein intake moderate on *TSC*.

There is a term you should be familiar with in order to understand why or how protein is converted into sugar: gluconeogenesis. Gluconeogenesis provides all the glucose you need to restore thyroid function. The body uses gluconeogenesis when it breaks down proteins into sugar. This occurs mainly in the liver. So, if glucose is running low in the blood, the body simply takes the proteins we are feeding it and turns them into sugar (in the absence of carbohydrates).

I'm not getting all "scientific" on you!!! I simply want to explain why it's important to keep protein moderate and not worry about not consuming enough carbs!

Here's an example of life before and after *TSC*. When I was bulimic and starving myself, my blood sugar levels were out of control. They were

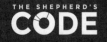

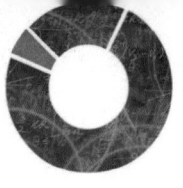
not stable. I would eat jellybeans for breakfast, a scone for lunch, and nothing for dinner. I was putting pure refined sugar into my bloodstream, and this would wreak havoc on my glucose levels and cause hunger pangs.

Now, as a believer in and proponent of *TSC System*, I eat moderate amounts of protein, lots and lots of good fat and only minimal carbs, and I feel completely satiated and energized all day long. It's been like night and day.

Finding *TSC* removed this phenomenon of craving that I experienced every day of my life for years. Now that I'm eating differently than I was, I can focus on the important things in my life and be fully present. It freed me from my food addiction permanently, transformed my overall health and fitness, and allowed me to focus on family, friends, and my relationship with my healthy self.

Believe me, it can do the same for you... if you take a leap of faith and let it work a miracle in your life, as it has in mine and so many others.

> *So Jesus said to him, "Unless you see signs and wonders you will not believe."*
>
> ***John 4:48***

 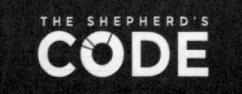

IT'S YOUR CHOICE – CHOOSE WISELY

Sometimes, our drug of choice (in this case, it's sugar and carbs) becomes our best friend. They become everything to us and making them go away or getting rid of them can be really heart-breaking and gut wrenching.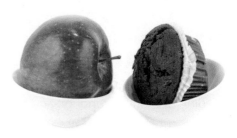

However, a good question to ask yourself is, how much do you value your health? Do you want to lose weight, feel better, and live longer? Do you want to see your kids graduate and get married?

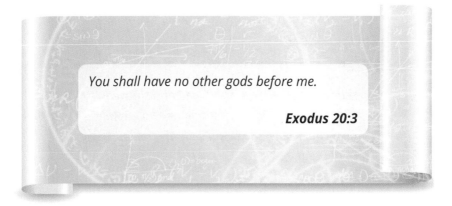

You shall have no other gods before me.

Exodus 20:3

 If you want to be healthy and avoid cardiovascular complications that come with eating sugar and carbs, and if you want to avoid chronic fatigue, pain, stroke, Parkinson's, Alzheimer's, or other illnesses that can set in because your body's not in a state of health, then read and follow *TSC System*.

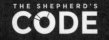

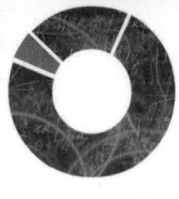

I think that most of us can say that when we wake up everything hurts, we're still tired, feel bloated and have no color in our faces or no radiant, healthy glow. But these very symptoms can motivate us to throw out the junk—the food that's been hurting us all these years.

The choice is simple, but doing it can be hard; it can be like saying goodbye to a good friend. It's the same thing as quitting smoking, stopping drinking alcohol or any drug. You're going to make friends with new substances that are helpful and good for you.

When you surrender and you admit that this substance or this food or whatever it is, has a hold on you, you say, "You know what, I can't control it or manage it anymore, I'm done. I'm giving it over to something greater than myself, namely a higher power."

> *Fear not, for I am with you; be not dismayed, for I am your God; I will strengthen you, I will help you, I will uphold you with my righteous right hand.*
>
> **Isaiah 41:10**

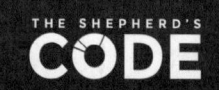

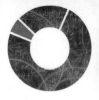

> When you make the decision to remove the trigger foods and replace them with the healthy foods that we are recommending with *TSC System*, you will feel free.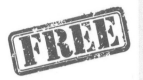

You'll feel happy, light and much better. It's truly an awakening. The mental clarity from eating this way is wonderful. No more brain fog, no more waking up with a food hangover. All those days are over once you embrace this new way of eating. Utilizing *TSC* can result in feeling **the best you have ever felt in your life**. That's a pretty big deal.

After my son Luke was born, I felt horrible about my physical self. I saw and felt rolls on my stomach. At night, Luke would be on my chest as I was feeding him, and I would count the rolls. I thought, "Oh, my God, I've never had rolls on my stomach in my life. This is so foreign and so uncomfortable." I was kind of scared. I thought, "Am I ever going to be able to get my body back? I hadn't worked out, and when I got on the scale, I thought the scale was broken. I really believed there was no way that number could be me.

I went to Bed, Bath and Beyond and bought another scale, a high-tech, fancy scale. When I got home, I stepped on it, and the numbers were the same. I was really freaking out; I was panicked. I was at my wits end. I wanted to be able to play with my son and be a healthy mom, run around, play catch, play football, and do all the things that little boys love to do, but part of me thought, "There are women out there that are chubby and overweight, but still attractive. Maybe I could just be like one of them," and I kept thinking of Delta Burke. At one point,

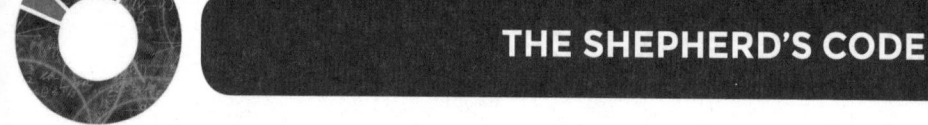
she was Miss America, and then she put on so much weight, but, to me, she still looked attractive. I was considering trying to be a chubby mom, accepting myself at that weight and shape.

I thought that not only my exercise but also my food plan would have to change. I couldn't just eat whatever I wanted with the excuse, "Well, I'm eating for two." I knew that I had to get back on track... I knew exactly what to eat because I had been eating "healing fats" for years.

I just had to get back on track. I began a workout regimen, and I was strict with my food as *TSC* says to be, with minimal carbs, moderate protein, and high fat. I was back in my regimen the way I had been all those years prior to Luke coming into my life. It took about three months; then, I saw amazing results. I was back down to a size four. I felt healthy and strong, and I looked fit and lean.

I looked better than I did before I had Luke.

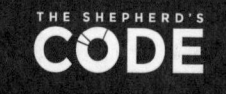

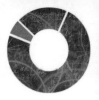

STEP 3: GET STARTED ON THE IDEAL YOU

I am sure, like me, that you want to be the ideal version of yourself. You want to be the ideal weight, feel good, and have everything fall into place with energy and confidence, but you have no idea where to start or how to begin this endeavor to become the ideal you.

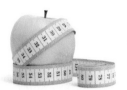

Are you ready to make the transformation? This chapter will show you exactly how to do it with Step 3 of *The Shepherd's Code*.

I know how you feel. You may doubt that it is even possible for you. You've tried things before, and they didn't work. You'd like to get results like mine; you'd like to be an ideal version of yourself, but you don't know how to get started, and you need a simple plan.

You may even doubt that you're worth investing the time and energy it takes to become a different person. Sometimes, it's so much easier to give up, to just give up. It's easy, yes, but don't you want to take the challenge of becoming the ideal you, with health and vigor? Do you want to be able to play with your kids, ride a bike, shoot hoops and really be involved?

You may have a lot of doubts about your ability to follow this diet and questions about exactly what to do. You might be asking, "Great, so what do I have to eat? Am I going to be hungry? Is it going to be awful? Am I going to feel deprived? Why should I bother?" I can relate to all those feelings because I have been in that situation. Some of you may think, "It's too hard, and I'm too old," or "Oh, I'm a grandparent. I'm a grand mom or a grand pop. I don't need to look so fabulous." Sometimes, it's not about looks. It's about physical health. You must trust the process....

Do you not know that you are God's temple and that God's Spirit dwells in you? If anyone destroys God's temple, God will destroy him. For God's temple is holy, and you are that temple.

1 Corinthians 3:16-17

Now, the question is, "How do you go about transforming into the ideal you?"

One of the things I utilized when I was getting started many moons ago was a three-day, quick start program, and this was simply something that I found in some research I did about getting started on TSC System. After the three days, you feel so great, you want to keep going, so it's like a jump start. You can begin your program by utilizing a three-day or a seven-day quick start plan.

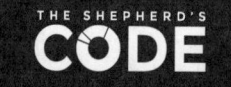
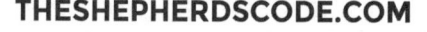

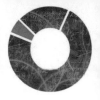

THE SHEPHERD'S CODE SYSTEM
3-DAY QUICK START:

DAY 1

 Breakfast:
- Cream Cheese Pancakes with butter and sugar-free syrup (if desired)
- coffee with heavy cream (& no-carb sweetener if desired)
- bacon or sugar-free breakfast sausage

How do you make Cream Cheese Pancakes? Simply take a cup of cream cheese and 2 or 3 eggs, add a dash of vanilla and blend in a blender! Cook in a pan, just like regular pancakes. Be sure to use butter (lots of butter) for your pan and pancakes once they are cooked... Delicious!!

Tip for making the best pancakes ever: Wait for the bubbles, exercise patience and wait for the bubbles to pop up under the entire pancake, then flip.

 Snack: 2-3 sticks of string cheese or a handful of almonds (salted)

 Lunch:
Ham and cheese rolled in Cream Cheese Pancakes with mayonnaise and arugula or spinach

 Snack: Half of an avocado with lite salt and pepper

 Dinner:
- Buffalo chicken wings
- High-fat blue cheese dressing
- Celery sticks

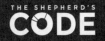

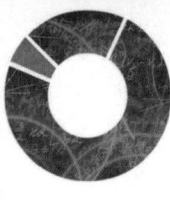

DAY 2

 Breakfast:
- Eggs (any style)
- bacon or sugar free sausage
- coffee with heavy cream (& no-carb sweetener if desired)

 **Snack:**
Half an avocado with salt and pepper or cheese sticks

 **Lunch:**
Simple tuna salad-tuna in water, mayonnaise or olive oil, salt and pepper, romaine lettuce leaves
Just spoon it in and eat like a taco.

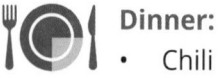 **Snack:**
Handful of almonds and/or 2 sticks of string cheese

 Dinner:
- Chili
- cheddar cheese, sour cream

How do you make TSC Chili? Brown ground beef in a pan with taco seasoning, add cheese and sour cream

 Dessert:
½ cup full-fat Greek yogurt with 1 tablespoon almond butter and 1 tablespoon cocoa. Delicious!

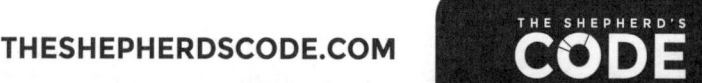

DAY 3

Breakfast:
- Cream Cheese Pancakes
- coffee with heavy cream (& no-carb sweetener if desired)
- bacon or sugar-free breakfast sausage

Snack: Handful of almonds and/or 2 sticks of string cheese

Lunch:
Leftover chili, tuna salad, or ham and cheese/pancake rollups

Snack:
1 cup chicken broth, half an avocado with lite salt and pepper

Dinner:
- Grilled lemon-chicken thighs
- Mashed cauliflower with cheddar cheese
- Salad with oil and vinegar and add bacon if you would like

In addition to the 3-day meal plan above, you will find 14 days of delicious breakfast, lunch and dinner meal plans in our member area, **shepcode.com/members**, and if you're not yet a member, you'll find all the information you need to join today.

The question is, "How do you go about transforming into your ideal?" It depends. You can begin transforming into the ideal you whether you are a person who likes to eat out all the time, or you order food in. Maybe you're a mom and a wife and you go food shopping frequently—you're always at the grocery store—there is a way for you to get started.

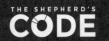

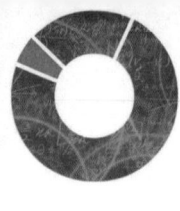
HERE IS A SAMPLE MENU
FROM RED ROBIN:

Clucks and Fries – NO

Prime Rib Dip – good choice without the bun

Arctic Cod Fish and Chips – NO

Buzz Clucks and Mac and Cheese – NO

Ensenada Chicken Platter – Good Choice substitute salad and veggies with cheese for potato and or fries

Clucks and shrimp – NO

Red's Nantucket Seafood Scatter (all fried) – NO

Red's Tavern Burger – Good choice without the bun... add bacon and cheese

Sautéed Shroom Burger – Good Choice without the bun

Bacon and Cheese Burger – Good choice without the bun

Bleu Ribbon Burger – Good choice without bun and onion straws

Guacamole Burger – Good choice without the bun

Wedgie Burger – BEST CHOICE, We have a winner!!!

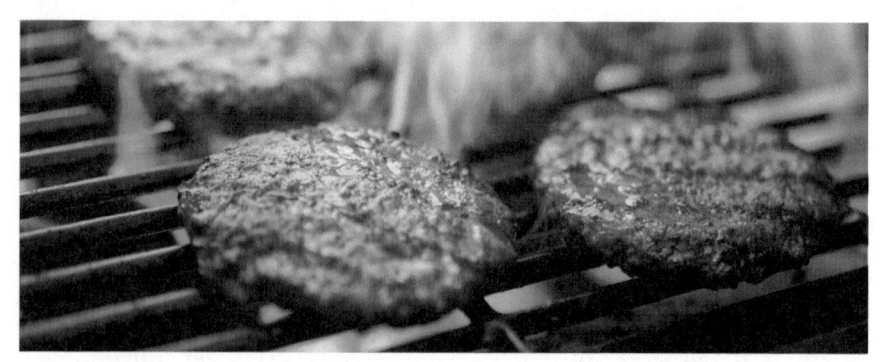

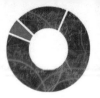

HELPFUL HINTS FOR GROCERY SHOPPING

1. Use the acronym HALT: Hungry, Angry, Lonely and Tired. If you are any one of these things, do not go grocery shopping! Wait until you have rested, eaten and or resolved the pressing issue.

2. Stay in the outer perimeter of the supermarket. Here you will find vegetables, eggs, meats, yogurt, butter, cheese and berries.

3. Read labels!! Carbs are everywhere!

4. Stick to the items on your list! Do not try to 'freestyle' shop!

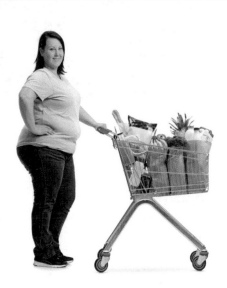

You are neither hopeless nor helpless, but it does pay to have a plan when you are first learning how to shop smart and transition away from the typical Western diet. The first thing to do is to have it set in your mind what you are looking for. Your objective is to find "healing fats". You'll find these fats come in many forms that will delight you as you fill your cart and consider all the delicious meals you have to look forward to.

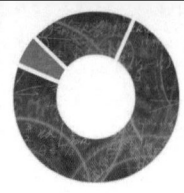
A NOTE ON COOKING METHODS

Vegetables are best enjoyed raw, grilled, or steamed but can always be topped with cheese, butter or olive oil for variety and satiety.

Frying is generally not recommended because it usually involves the use of a breading. However, by using something like parmesan cheese or macadamia nuts in place of breadcrumbs, you can still enjoy some of your favorite fried foods without risking your fat-burning potential.

Here is one example of a quick, easy and versatile recipe using our suggested breadcrumb alternative: Parmesan Crusted Scallops.

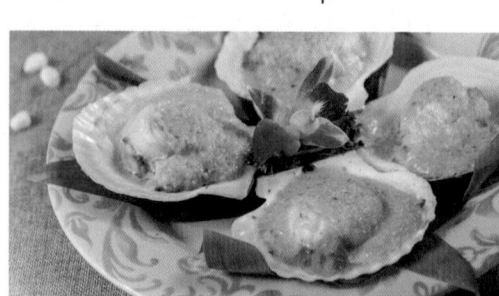

Parmesan Crusted Scallops
Ingredients:
- wild caught scallops
- Parmesan cheese
- 3 eggs
- butter

Preparation:
1. Heat skillet on medium-high and add butter.
2. Beat eggs in a bowl.
3. Grate Parmesan cheese into a separate bowl.
4. Rinse scallops and pat dry with a paper towel.
5. Dip scallops in eggs then dredge in grated cheese.
6. Carefully place scallops into skillet.
7. Cook until golden brown, about 2 minutes on each side

The same recipe may be applied to chicken or pork cutlets. Use a meat thermometer to check for doneness as cooking times will vary.

THE SHEPHERD'S
CODE

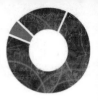

But whoever drinks of the water that I will give him will never be thirsty again. The water that I will give him will become in him a spring of water welling up to eternal life.

John 4:14

One way to to jazz up your drinking water is to add lemon juice, lime juice or fresh cucumber.

I also recommend Hint water found at the local grocery store. The Hints are carb free, sugar free, calorie free with hint of fruit flavoring.

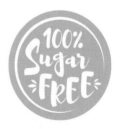

Remember to read all labels when you're not sure what's in the food or drink you are selecting from! Just because it says zero calories does not necessarily mean it has zero carbs!

What about food selection when your meals come on the run? You might be the type of person who either loves to eat out or has to for

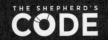

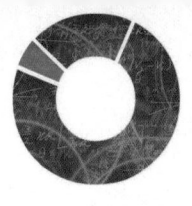

work related opportunities (or limitations, as the case may be). If you find yourself ordering food off of a menu on the regular, this next bit of advice will make sticking to a plan and achieving success a whole lot easier.

The key is to order meals focused around a protein. Look at the menu and decide if you're in the mood for chicken, fish or beef. Find a meal with that main ingredient then make a few substitutions that will cater to your tastes and dietary needs. For example, you could have a steak with steamed broccoli instead of mashed potatoes. Or, you might have a cup of green beans, smothered in butter, instead of french fries. Soup, salad, and grilled chicken can come together as an entire meal in itself anytime. Remember, this isn't an attempt at low calorie living; enjoy your favorite salad dressing and a cream soup if you so desire!

Avoid the temptation to order carb loaded sandwiches. If you love sandwiches, like I do, you can still order one, but either make that sandwich into a lettuce wrap or just take the bread off when it gets to your table. Try your waiter, and say, "I would like a ham and cheese melt without the bread." Most restaurants can accommodate such requests without a problem.

Now, I know many of you love dessert. You look forward to it. You might even eat less during the main meal to save room for dessert. Though it's tasty and addictive, one of the benefits of being on *TSC* is that you will lose your craving for dessert. You'll be enjoying the life-giving food you're eating so much that dessert will no longer seem like the icing on the cake.

However, if you're a person for whom sweets is less of an addiction and more of a way to balance the richness of your dinner, there are really tasty and healthful options that will build you up rather than take you down. One way to go is for berries and whipped cream. Yes, please!

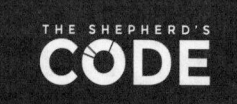

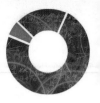

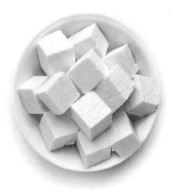

Or, if you'd rather, do as the Europeans do and close with an assortment of cheeses—cheese, not cheesecake!

Luckily, there is now an ice-cream that even fits the bill. It goes by the name of Halo Top. *TSC System* recommends it for a quick ice cream fix when you're at home. It only has a handful of carbs per half cup serving. Sorry, but any other ice cream will have you tripping over your halo in no time.

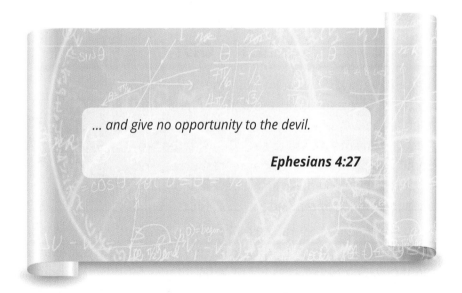

... and give no opportunity to the devil.

Ephesians 4:27

You do need to be careful with dessert because it can trigger so many temptations, but generally, when you are on *TSC System*, you are not going to want to eat sweets because your body will no longer crave that brain chemical reaction.

Another frequent pitfall comes once we walk through the doors of the movie theater. Popcorn can be hard to resist, at first. But corn is full of carbs and popping it doesn't change that. The same goes for those trays of nachos. Corn chips are no better than popcorn, and is it really fair to call that topping cheese? Pass! If you are already following a consistently keto diet and can afford to step away from it for a moment, mozzarella sticks or chicken nuggets can fit the bill as a popcorn substitute. Both are fairly low in carbs in relation to the rest of their ingredients.

LET'S GO!

To put it simply, if you enjoy your meals with the foods I've suggested and avoid the culprits that stand in the way of ketosis, you're going to see results. Like my mom used to say, "Get with the program!" *TSC* provides the guidance, resources, and support to help you make smart decisions and live a healthier more vibrant life.

RESULTS

If you are prepared for rapid results and astonishing transformation I have something special just for you. Your kind of eager commitment and motivation for success is just what it takes for driven individuals to see and feel results using a three-day quick start. My own journey following *TSC* began in this way and had me noticing measurable and lasting change in less than a week. I believe you can do it too!

The *Shepherds Code System* is a permanent solution to a temporary problem.

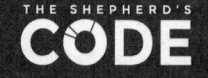

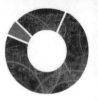

> *Blessed is the man who remains steadfast under trial, for when he has stood the test he will receive the crown of life, which God has promised to those who love him.*
>
> **James 1:12**

According to the Harvard School of Public Health, excess weight harms health in many ways. It increases the risk of developing conditions such as diabetes, heart diseases, osteoarthritis, and even some cancers. It can also reduce your lifespan. Treating obesity and other related conditions costs billions of dollars. By one estimate, the US spent 190 billion on obesity-related healthcare expenses.

Let me tell you about how I was able to first accept the reality of my excess weight and then transform it... and next, how it changed my life.

It was one fateful day many years ago after having my son, when I got on the scale and had to admit that my weight was not healthy. Then and there I accepted the situation for what it was. I knew that I had to make a change, and determined to claim my body back after having had a baby. My mind was set and from then on there was no turning back.

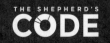

In much the same way, If you decide to utilize *TSC*, I guarantee that you will look and feel amazing. Your energy will be through the roof, and if you are like me, when you successfully lose weight you may have more confidence in your abilities and self-worth. You'll gain control of things like cravings and be able to manage all of the other symptoms that go along with unstable blood sugar.

> It's up to you. Either you will become the ideal you, or you won't. Isn't that the truth for all of us?

If you don't change to this new way of eating, you can expect the same symptoms: fatigue, pain, heart burn, bloating, irritability, and the list goes on! If nothing changes, nothing changes. If you don't try, you won't have success. Your life won't differ much from what it is now. You'll be inside your comfort zone, but I guarantee you this: You will never be the ideal you. To taste the fruit, we've got to test the limb! I promise you, the limb won't break!

I had no choice when my limb to test was set before me.

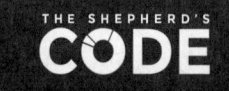

STEP 4:
REST AND EAT RIGHT

My husband was brain dead. I was numb. I was thinking, "How am I going to carry on? How am I going to live? How am I going to even do life now that he is gone?" My husband was diagnosed with ALS three years prior to that day.

For three years I had been his sole caregiver and best friend. I made sure that he was okay in any way that I could. I took care of him day in and day out, as well as my little boy, who was then only five years old. It was exhausting, but that's what wives do.

That's what you do as an honorable wife and loving mother.

His systems broke down, one by one. He couldn't speak. He couldn't walk well. He couldn't do anything that he used to do on his own. He couldn't even shave. Although his mind was perfectly intact, his body was slowly but surely falling apart.

The day my husband was pronounced brain dead was the final goodbye. I was undone. I hadn't eaten in three days. I was bone-fatigued. I was tired and depressed. Well, tired is an understatement. I was exhausted. I could barely walk. I couldn't even drive myself to the hospital. That evening, when I went home after I said goodbye to my husband, I was praying. I couldn't think of anything else to do but to pray.

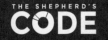

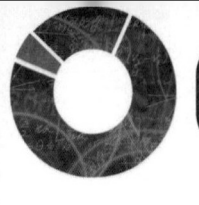
> *Likewise the Spirit helps us in our weakness. For we do not know what to pray for as we ought, but the Spirit himself intercedes for us with groanings too deep for words.*
>
> **Romans 8:26**

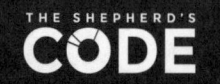

I realized I needed to take care of myself. It was that or just die. In my grief and desperation I had stopped following *TSC* for a moment that stretched into a few days. I couldn't eat. I couldn't swallow. Just the thought of food was revolting. Not only that, but, my brain fog had returned. I couldn't think straight. I was frazzled; I was undone.

With what little brainpower that remained, I realized something. I thought, "If I can't chew, and the thought of meat and vegetables is not a palatable solution right now, why don't I make shakes?"

There are many shakes that fulfill the requirements of *TSC*. They're useful, helpful, and easy. They nourish you in the way your body needs to be nourished.

I started making some wonderfully nutritious shakes that were filled with good fats and protein. They helped me to maintain a healthy weight to face this very emotional and difficult time.

Using well-chosen snacks and shakes that contained the "healing fats" that we've been discussing, like coconut oil, olive oil and almonds, I was able to incorporate all the nutrition I needed.

That helped not only with weight management but also to conquer the unbelievable fatigue and brain fog. I once again had energy and felt so much better.

The shakes you'll find in *TSC* were especially instrumental in getting me to the point where I could maintaining my healthy weight, clarity, and energy. They kept me functioning as I was supposed to, the way God designed me to.

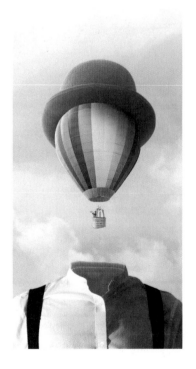

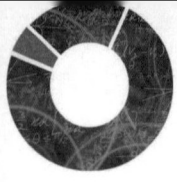
FIND A WAY

We are a nation of people who are busy, overweight, and dealing with the many heavy realities of a fallen world. Unfortunately, that just the norm. We experience an onslaught of daily events that cause stress: death, tests, public failure, fear, divorce, who knows what. Sometimes, these difficult times aren't even all that hard to take in stride, but when lumped together, life can get hairy! Add to that the weight of raising children and keeping God's will a priority, and the load seems almost unbearable. Yet, He promises:

> *No temptation has overtaken you that is not common to man. God is faithful, and he will not let you be tempted beyond your ability, but with the temptation he will also provide the way of escape, that you may be able to endure it.*
>
> **1 Corinthians 10:13**

Life is an immeasurable blessing that is really neither black nor white. It's one of those "whole ball of wax" things. With an ever constant flow of positive and negative moments shaping our existence, it really is easy to veer off our diet, our food plan, or our self-care. Without even noticing at first, we just slip away from it.

 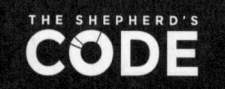

I fully relate to the feeling of having to constantly dodge curveballs; but I'm here to show you that it can be done with grace and a growing sense of acceptance as you learn to navigate difficult times with the wisdom, clarity, and self-respect that comes from becoming your healthy best.

> *Beloved, I pray that all may go well with you and that you may be in good health, as it goes well with your soul.*
>
> **John 1:2**

Let me take you back some years to a time when I was living in New York. I was three years out of rehab working as a missionary in New York City. That type of work was so mentally, physically, and spiritually exhausting that today I look back on it so very grateful that I had *TSC System* to keep me strong. I relied heavily on the snacks because a lot of times I'd be without access to food. I was out in the field for eight or ten hours at a time, so I would bring food with me. It was easy and simple. It kept me level, and in tune with the work that I needed to do there. It was a prime opportunity for me to learn how important it was to take care of myself so that I could take care of others.

It's like when on a plane they go over the preflight emergency landing instructions. They say, "Ladies and gentlemen, if you're sitting near a child, please take care to secure your own mask before trying to help

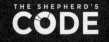

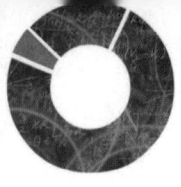
them with theirs." They say it because if we as caretakers run out of oxygen, we're helpless and so are those who rely on us. What good is that? You need to self-care, put your oxygen mask on so you're able to help others. If you don't take care of yourself, you can't help anybody else. Even when it's hard, you can dig deep and find your source of strength. We all have access if we ask for it.

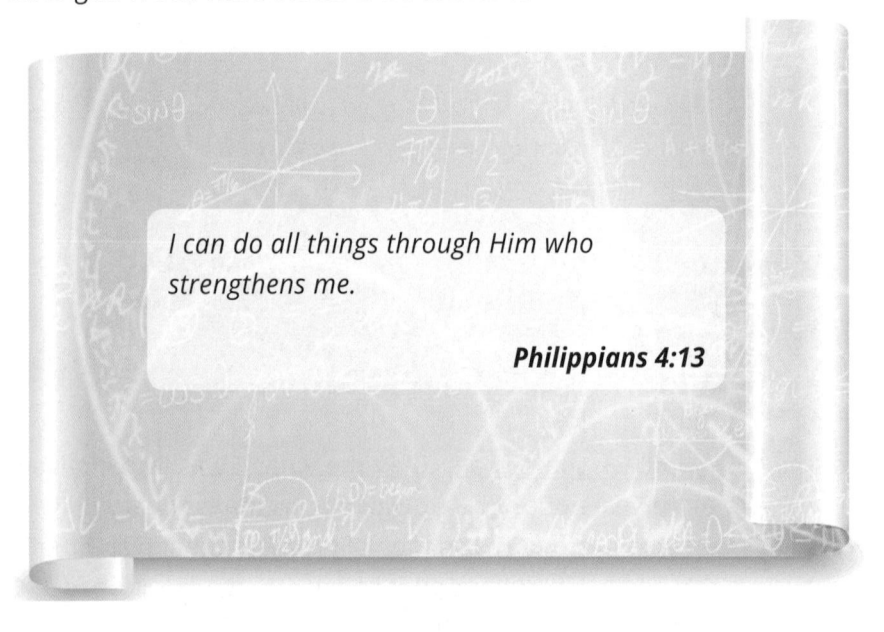

I can do all things through Him who strengthens me.

Philippians 4:13

Even if you don't know it yet, I want you to hear and begin to believe that food is not your enemy. It's your friend. Food is instrumental in self-care. It is what God has blessed us with to stay healthy and strong.

If you stick with *TSC System* in times of stress and anxiety and when you're exhausted in life, as I did in New York and when my husband was dying, you'll be able to manage these times much more effectively than you would be if you were not utilizing food in a proper way.

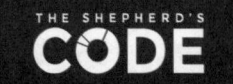

If you do use *TSC System* in times of stress, you won't find yourself gaining or losing dozens of pounds at a time. It is possible to stay strong and healthy at all times. It's all about putting your trust in the One who made you and using His gifts to care for yourself.

If you decide not to utilize *TSC* in times of stress, like through divorce or loss of a job, or even during exciting times, such as when you get married, you can expect to feel terrible. Stress is a killer. It can kill you quickly with a heart attack, or slowly with other things like chronic fatigue or eating disorders. It can cause skin rashes, pain, and digestive issues. It can even cause cancer. It can make any existing condition much worse.

Stress is inevitable, so being prepared for it is a good idea. *The Shepherd's Code* can help you during those times.

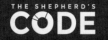

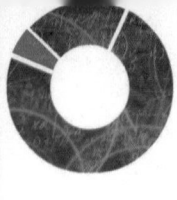

STEP 5:
RESIST TEMPTATION

TEMPTING FOOD

In Chapter Five, we are going to discuss how to resist temptation.

Temptation lurks around every corner. Foods and drink tempt us. Friends and family members who still don't understand what it is and why we're following *The Shepherd's Code* tempt us. This is not a lost cause. We will discuss strategies that will help us stand strong in the face of temptation throughout this chapter.

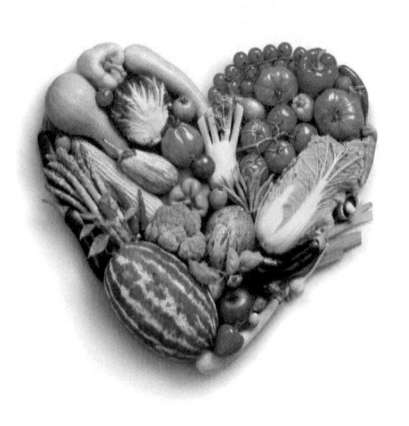

I can't say that I've always been strong. Not even starting *TSC* was enough to made me strong in the beginning. I used to cry in the supermarket. I mean, of all places, there I was, bawling my eyes out, terrified. In a supermarket, long after I got on *TSC*, I would cry sometimes because I feared that I might fail to resist temptation, that I would fall off the wagon and go back to my unhealthy lifestyle. For many long years, food was my enemy, and it was a frightening enemy at times.

There was one incident that stands out in my memory. It was about three years after rehab and two years into my *TSC* recovery. There I was in New York City, in an unfamiliar place. I was in a supermarket with

 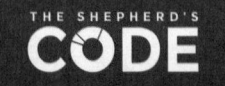

tempting food all around. I didn't know exactly where everything was in this new place, so I was a little anxious.

I had been sick for so long, and even though I was well on the road to recovery, I still had this fear that I might fall off the wagon. I felt like an alcoholic who knew that one drink could ruin everything. I could sabotage my recovery if I weren't strong and able to give my will over to my higher power.

How did I handle what amounted to a panic attack in a public place? I opened my TSC Toolbox and created a mantra.

It goes like this: "One moment at a time." I've used that mantra for a very long time now, and it works like a charm.

> *Be anxious for nothing, but in everything by prayer and supplication, with thanksgiving, let your requests be made known to God; and the peace of God, which surpasses all understanding, will guard your hearts and minds through Christ Jesus.*
>
> ***Philippians 4:6-7***

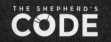

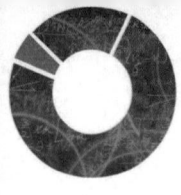

THE SHEPHERD'S CODE TOOLBOX

I'm sure you too know how tempting certain foods can be, especially the sugary sweet donuts, cookies and candy stacked in the inner aisles of almost any supermarket. They have no nutritional value and are not on *TSC System* food plan, but they smell and taste great and are packaged to tempt you into indulging yourself at any cost.

It's a common problem, but you can and will resist the temptation to buy and eat these unhealthy foods if you keep your *TSC* Toolbox handy and use it whenever the pressure is on.

> The *The Shepherd's Code* Toolbox includes **five useful tools and strategies for resisting temptation:**

1. Flee. When tempted, think of the word "flee." Allow yourself to simply walk away, take a moment and pause, breathe, and regroup. It only takes 90 seconds for the brain to shift in its thinking, so all you need to do is redirect your mind. It helps so much.

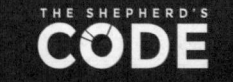

2. Breathe and clear your mind. Whether it's in the supermarket, at a restaurant, or out at a party, before you walk into a place where there may be temptation, take a few deep breaths and clear your mind. Then ask yourself if you want to do the things you may be tempted by. Decide ahead of time what your priorities are. Then the answer will be easy. Falling into temptation is never worth it.

> *Watch and pray that you may not enter into temptation. The spirit indeed is willing, but the flesh is weak.*
>
> **Matthew 26:41**

3. Call a trusted friend.

> *Two people are better off than one, for they can help each other succeed.*
>
> **Ecclesiastes 4:9**

Lean on someone who understands your situation and wants the best for you, someone who is abreast of what you're going through and understands your feelings. You will feel much better in minutes, just talking about your apprehension.

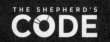

4. Try Ketostix. Ketostix are tiny urine test-sticks that you can buy at Walgreens or any supermarket. They're cheap and come 50 to a pack. If the stick changes color even slightly, you have proof that you are burning fat instead of sugar. When you are on *TSC System*, that's proof that you're doing the right thing. Seeing something tangible like that helps you to stay on track because you don't want to mess it up. This is motivating because it is evidence of your hard work. It is evidence that all your efforts of staying on this food plan are paying off and encourages you to stay the path.

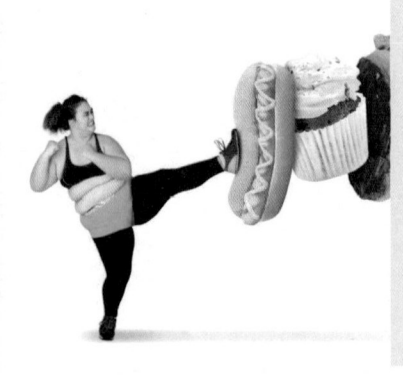

Once you've adapted to fat burning by resisting tempting foods, and seen proof of your progress with the Ketostix, you'll know that your body is burning fat instead of sugar and glucose. And, guess what. Once you've turned your body on to being a fat-melting machine, you **won't want to turn it off**.

TEMPTING DRINKS

After I had Luke, I started eating the *The Shepherd's Code* way and working out again, but I wasn't seeing the results I wanted. I was extremely upset about my weight, how I was feeling and looking. My weight had plateaued. So, I hired a trainer, with whom I worked out at least five times a week. I had decided that I was on a mission. I really wanted my body back quickly.

There I was, alone and caring for a baby. I had no job, no friends. I had just moved to a new state, and was still getting used to being married. I had a new baby to take care and time enough to be alone with my thoughts most of the time.

To fill that void, I started drinking wine. I'd be preparing dinner, and I would have the bottle open and pour myself a nice glass of wine. I thought, "Oh, it's three o'clock. It's okay to drink. It's late enough." I would start drinking wine just to feel a little bit better.

When I said, "Hey, my weight plateaued, I'm not seeing the results I want," my trainer asked me, "What's going on? Are you drinking alcohol?" I said, "Yes," and he asked me how often. I said, "Oh, just with dinner."

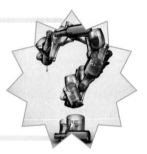

He said, "Do you eat dinner every day?" I said, "Yes," so then he said, "Kristina, you might as well just go home now. If you're going to continue to drink every single day and come here, you're throwing away your money because alcohol can stop your weight loss."

Alcohol can sabotage your weight loss and throw you right out of the fat-burning phase. The liver's job is to metabolize fat. When we ingest alcohol, the liver gets to work helping the kidneys flush out those toxins. Therefore, it is unable to do its primary job of metabolizing fat. This has nothing to do with calories!

I decided to put the alcohol down for one month. After 30 days, the weight just fell off.

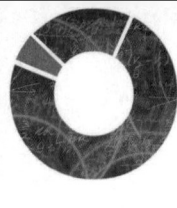

DRINK THE SPIRIT INSTEAD

I know that you want to look great. A lot of people would love to look great without giving up wine, beer, or cocktails, but the truth is, alcohol will sabotage your weight loss. Why? Because wine metabolizes into sugar. But there's another reason. It's not just about the calories. As I said before, the job of our kidneys is to get rid of toxins. The liver metabolizes fat. When we drink alcohol, the liver must help the kidneys. The liver can't do its job of metabolizing fat if it has toxins from wine and beer flooding the system.

The Shepherd's Code does not require you to stop drinking completely, but it does call for moderation, and this is important, especially during the first 30 days of *The Shepherd's Code*.

One of the tools I frequently use to deal with temptation from alcohol is a mantra. The mantra I use is, "Nothing tastes as good as abstinence (from alcohol) feels!" This mantra really helps because I feel amazing when eating the way *The Shepherd's Code* recommends.

I don't want to lose the feeling of high energy and mental clarity. Knowing I am doing the right thing regarding food and alcohol is also comforting. I feel safe in my own skin! Why would you want to sabotage your own well being with cocktails? It's like trading feeling great for headaches, dehydration and anxiety! It just doesn't make sense.

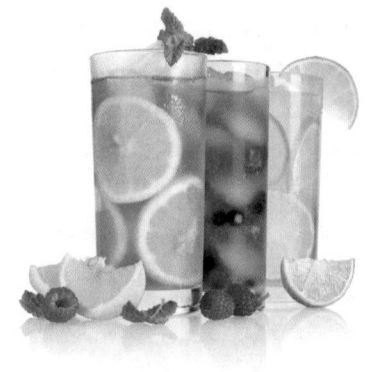

Another tool you can use when tempted by alcohol is to FLEE! You can simply walk away, leave, vamoose, scram or exit the building! You may be thinking, "People will think I'm crazy if I do that."

If what others think is more important to you than your health, that's another problem to address. You must begin to put yourself first at times (self-care) to stay healthy! Remember, moderation is key.

> When I want to have a drink, I choose wisely. My favorite cocktail is vodka, club soda and lime over lots of ice.

It tastes delicious and has zero carbs and zero sugar. I sip it slowly, and one drink can last a couple of hours. I can socialize, mingle, attend parties, celebrate and remain in the fat burning phase metabolically with a drink that has zero carbs!

Another trick I use when socializing or out to dinner is to always order a glass of water with lemon. The water helps you remain hydrated while consuming alcohol. It also looks like a cocktail and feels like a cocktail in your hand. You don't have to feel awkward or "different" just because you are choosing not to drink excessively!

I have noticed that many restaurants are acknowledging people's focus on health by offering drinks made with Truvia or stevia instead of sugar. For example, one day recently, I was out to lunch with a girlfriend. I was celebrating the release and success of my new book. I decided to treat myself and order a cocktail. The menu offered a mojito made with stevia, vodka, mint leaves and lime. I was so excited! Instead of drinking something loaded with sugar and carbs, I indulged in this amazing sugar-free, carb-free mojito!! It was a delightful cocktail!

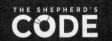

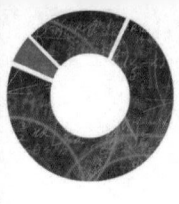
It's important to be vigilant with alcohol, but after a while, you will find that you no longer crave it or even desire it in the same way. I believe the primary reason I was craving white wine years ago was blood sugar.

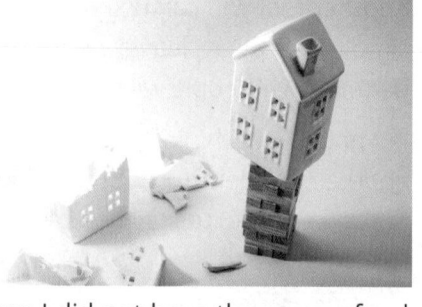

My blood sugar was so unstable; when I did not have the proper food plan, I would crave sugar to satisfy the craving. White wine was the ideal solution, so I thought.

I no longer have cravings because my blood sugar is stable. It's amazing how our bodies respond when we feed them properly!

TEMPTING SITUATIONS

I've also had to resist temptation to stop following *The Shepherd's Code* in situations involving family, friends and acquaintances, the times when pressure was applied with love or the best of intentions. I'm sure you've found yourself in similar situations.

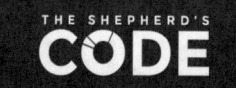

> *No temptation has overtaken you except what is common to mankind. And God is faithful; he will not let you be tempted beyond what you can bear. But when you are tempted, he will also provide a way out so that you can endure it.*
>
> **1 Corinthians 10:13**

When I would go home to visit my family during the holidays—Christmas, for example, my mother would say, "You can have just one, right? Are you still on that diet? You're still on it?"

My mother is Italian, and as such, she is very focused on food. That's true for many ethnic groups, so you too may be familiar with this mentality. Food and family, family and food, they go together.

My mom was in shock that I wouldn't eat a sugary dessert or a Christmas cookie that she had made. That was tough because I didn't want to let my mother down. I felt like I was letting her down if I didn't eat her sweets. You may feel that pressure from your family. Be prepared; they may be upset that you're not eating what they've made or what they want you to eat. But it's okay. We're doing this together. We're making the choices that will give us more holidays with family in the long run.

You just stay gentle with them and say, "You know, it really helps me be healthy. I appreciate, of course, that you made this for me." You can simply be kind and say no.

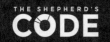

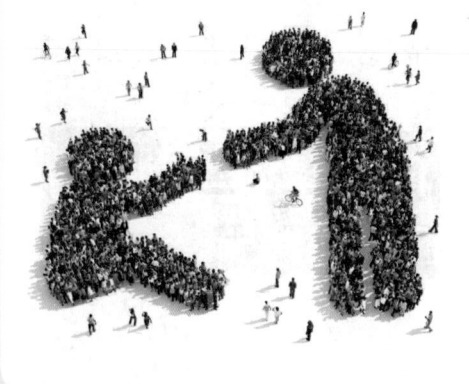

Similarly, when I went to visit my aunt recently, she hadn't seen me in a couple of years, and she looked at me and said, "What happened to you? Are you okay? Are you sick?"

I thought, "Oh boy, here we go."

You get so fit and so lean, looking great, that people sometimes think, "Are you still doing that old behavior?" She thought maybe I was still not eating or over-exercising and, in reality, I absolutely was not. I was eating healthy and working out in moderation.

Then, there's the unique pressure to eat and drink in unhealthy ways when you're on a date and want things to go smoothly. You don't know the person well, but you think he's just fabulous, or she's amazing, and you don't want to ruffle feathers or make them question who they thought you were. You want to have a nice time, and you worry that your date may think there is something wrong with you for declining alcohol or sweets (even in moderation).

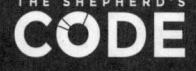

I remember one particular evening when I accepted a date with a handsome, successful guy. He took me to a fancy, expensive restaurant and ordered a bottle of wine. I knew I shouldn't have any, but I said, "Sure, why not? I'll have a glass of wine." In that moment I gave in because I wanted to please this person, but it didn't take me long to realize that this was not a wise decision. It wasn't worth damaging my health. **The next day, I felt awful!**

Well, I got right back on *TSC* and, when I saw him again, I said "You know what? That wine is not for me. I'm choosing not to drink today." He was perfectly fine with it.

I've since learned that you must speak your truth in situations like that where you feel tempted to eat or drink something that you know is not a wise choice for your health. If I had had the *TSC* Toolbox during this time in my life, I would have ordered a glass of water, paused a few minutes, and then either said, "No, thank you" to the wine, or I would have ordered a vodka and soda with lime. The situation would not have made me flinch! You now have tools to take with you into any place where food or alcohol may be tempting.

The whole point of me telling that story about my failure to stick to the *TSC System* is to encourage you not to give up if you make a mistake. We all do it from time to time, and it's not the end of the world. You haven't blown it completely. You can easily get right back on the plan. It's important to remember that you have choices. You can choose to sacrifice your health to please someone else, or you can choose to self-care, regardless of what people may think.

When we care for ourselves by setting boundaries with food and alcohol and people, we are protecting ourselves. Boundaries are like skin; they keep us from spilling out all over the place!

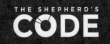

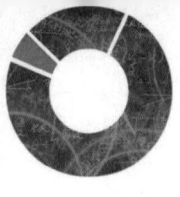
TEMPTATIONS BE GONE!

If you decide not to use the toolbox to resist temptation with *TSC*, you will kick yourself out of the fat-burning phase. That's discouraging, and your body will take longer to get the results that you're looking for.

There are people (I used to be one of them many years ago), that if they screw up or fall off the wagon, they never get back on. It happens for lots of us: We get so discouraged, so fed up, so tired and mad at ourselves that we decide, "Oh, forget it. I screwed up, and I'm not going to continue with this. It's just too hard."

The enemy wants us to fail. His job is to kill, steal and destroy our happiness and our lives. If we decide not to utilize the Toolbox to resist temptation while doing *TSC*, the enemy wins. He wins and plants that seed of doubt in so many people, the self-doubt. They ask themselves, "Am I strong enough? Am I worthy enough to do this?" That is all part of the defeatist plan to keep us off track and to keep us off balance.

If you use the tools in the Toolbox to resist temptation while doing *The Shepherd's Code*, you will find that you are succeeding and that you have more energy. You'll feel better, look better and become the person that you want to be. Using these tools keeps you from falling off the wagon. It's like putting on your oxygen mask before assisting the person next to you.

You may not think you're the kind of person who can resist temptation from foods you love, drinks you love, and friends and family who put pressure on you. You may think that you're always going to stumble because you always have, but if you use *The Shepherd's Code* Toolbox and you apply it in your life, you will discover that you are mentally and physically capable of resisting temptation and becoming the ideal you with *The Shepherd's Code*. And when you know that you can resist temptation on *The Shepherd's Code*, you're ready to take Step 6–Claim It. The next chapter will show you how to do just that!

 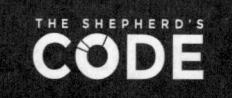

STEP 6:
CLAIM IT

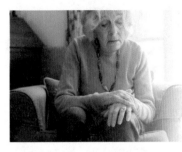

"Today I was diagnosed with Parkinson's," she said, and she knew her life would never be the same. When I met Dianna, she was a successful family lawyer. She and her husband practiced law together, and she had seen one of my ads in a local magazine.

She said, "Your ad says you can help people like me, people with Parkinson's. That you can help me have a better quality of life." She talked about the day she was diagnosed and the emotions she felt. It was hard for her, but she was on a mission to deal with the disease and do what she could to help herself.

My ad in a magazine called Quality Connections said, "Parkinson's, MS, ALS, I can help you with these crippling diseases. I'm a certified Corrective Exercise Specialist.

I'm a certified trainer and I have over 20 years' experience, so please call me. I can also help you with diet and nutritional needs."

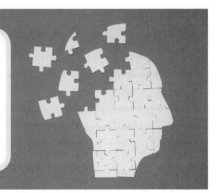

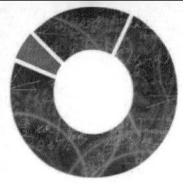
I believe many people would have given up at this point, but Dianna was not a quitter. I reminded her of a biblical story about two farmers. They were both praying for rain, but only one of them prepared for rain. He got the fields ready as if it were going to rain. He believed it so deeply that he just took it for granted that it was going to rain and plowed the fields, planted the seeds, and did everything that you do before rain comes.

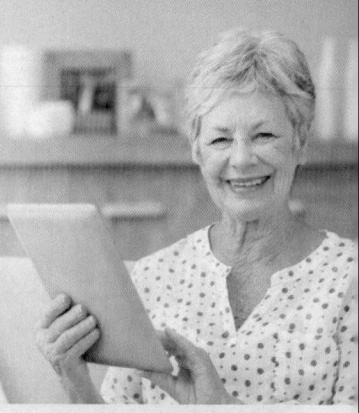

 Dianna is one of those people. She is preparing for rain. She's expecting to feel better, get better, and have a stronger quality of life, even with this disease, Parkinson's.

Dianna and I began working together. We trained two times a week for an hour: We did cardio, weight training and interval training. We still do. We did a lot of stretching and some yoga poses to help her get centered. As we were doing all this, Dianna was also following *The Shepherd's Code*. She was willing to change her food plan. She knew she had to because she was really overweight.

She was eating sugar in all forms: donuts, packaged goods, and processed foods; she really had no knowledge of nutrition and how it was affecting her. But when she got this disease, she knew she had to make significant changes.

She had a thriving law practice with her husband. She practiced family law, so she was very busy. She made lots of money and enjoyed her job a great deal. She told me she was angry that she got diagnosed with Parkinson's.

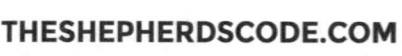

I reminded her of the story about the farmers and the rain. I said, "Wow. You're like the one who prepared for rain." She started laughing and said,

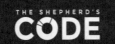

"Yes. I am not a quitter, and I'll do whatever it takes to get well." She started *TSC System*. She was doing Step One and she didn't even realize it. She was getting *TSC* mindset, wrapping her arms around, "Hey, I can eat delicious "healing fats", and I'm going to let go of these certain carbs and sugar," and she was believing that it would work if she did this. She definitely had a food addiction. She admitted that herself.

Dianna asked me a lot of questions about *TSC System* and whether certain fats are bad for you. She was so misinformed. I gave her several case studies of people who were overweight, followed this diet, lost the weight and have kept it off for years. Then I told her that *TSC* is recommended for her disease.

I educated her about what's going on when you eliminate carbs, and how the body responds. She was really excited. She looked up articles and bought books on low-carb diets and things of that nature, just to educate herself about what she would be doing.

She was able to jump right into Step Two and free herself from the food addiction because, when she began eating the food recommended on *TSC*, all her cravings disappeared. The sugar cravings, the carb cravings, everything just disappeared. She was so excited. She said, "You're not going to believe this. I didn't even think about donuts today." We would just laugh, but I said "That's why it works so well because you're rarely, if ever, hungry, and it helps eliminate those ups and downs in your blood sugar."

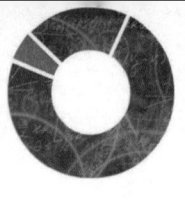
Dianna was really excited to jump in because she is a go-getter and not a quitter, and she thought, "Wow, I have Parkinson's, that's pretty extreme." Even if this food plan seemed extreme to her at first because it was different from what she was used to, she was willing to try it. I gave her the grocery list and a few sample days just to look at, and she decided to do a three-day "quick start."

> Her husband took her food shopping. She had the list with her; she bought everything she needed and even mapped out the seven days and what she would need for each day. Again, she was prepared to do this exactly the way you're supposed to. She was extremely successful.

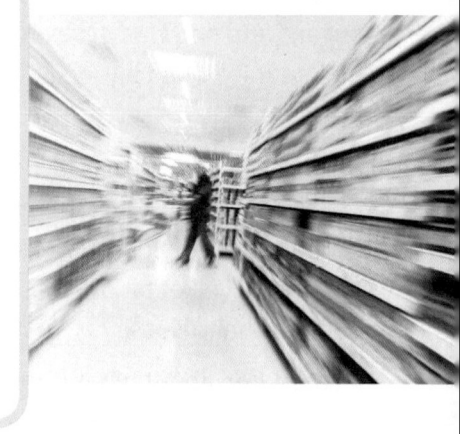

She took snacks with her to hold her over. She brought them with her everywhere, and she brought her lunch to work.

Her husband David was supportive. He took her food shopping, of course, because her dyskinesia (shaking) was very bad, so she was afraid to drive. She would shake all the time, and she couldn't control it. At first, the medication was not helping.

She was afraid to drive because if she had a quick spasm, she could veer off the road. Her husband took her wherever she needed to go to get all the items to begin the diet the right way.

 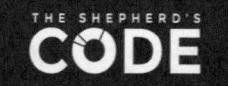

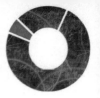

Without even knowing it, Dianna was going through the steps, just the way you're supposed to. She didn't even realize she was taking the necessary steps for her new lifestyle. Step Four was to rest and eat right.

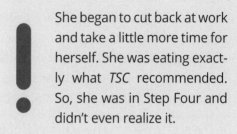

She began to cut back at work and take a little more time for herself. She was eating exactly what *TSC* recommended. So, she was in Step Four and didn't even realize it.

Her attitude was, "Look, I'm going to do this." And she just went for it. She knocked out the first four steps right away.

Dianna is absolute proof: You can develop the mindset, you can free yourself from addiction, you can get started on the seven-day plan or the three-day plan, and you can commit to resting and eating right all at once.

I presented Dianna with the steps and gave her a brief description of each step. She was in two or three steps at the same time. She began to rest and eat right and develop her *TSC* mindset all at the same time.

Dianna was committed and ready to claim it. When you're ready to claim it, you can quickly knock out the steps. That's what she did. Dianna had a disease that was crippling and shocking, but she was so ready to make those changes that Steps One through Four happened without any extra effort at all.

Having a disease is one example of a catalyst for change. You don't need a disease like Parkinson's to make these changes and to zip through Steps One through Four. You need the determination, the will, and the desire. Something I always say to my clients is, "Well, how badly do you want it? How badly do you want to be free of the fatigue, free of the weight, free of the 'I can't fit in a normal size car, I can't sit at the movies or on a plane'." Success depends on how badly you want it. That is the bottom line.

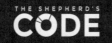

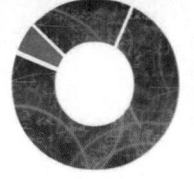
Step Five, which is to resist temptation, came automatically for Dianna because she was always prepared. She always had a snack with her; she always had a lunch with her so she was never so ravenous or out-of- control hungry that she'd turn to the vending machine or fall prey to a donut. She didn't do any of those things. She told me that when she went food shopping, she utilized the mental picture of letting her health go in first.

In the supermarket, she was solid, but the pressure of friends and family caused her some angst and concern. Even so, she was blunt and bold about her health, her needs and why she was doing this diet. She was very honest, and if she had to pause and walk away, that's what she did. She didn't care what they thought.

Dianna was considered obese. She did not drink. She never cared for it, she said. She may have a glass of wine on a special occasion, maybe once a year, but she gave that up as well. She didn't have any desire for it, so that part was easy. Alcohol was not a temptation for her. When it came to her workplace, she always had her food there, so she was fine. That's how she dealt with Step Five.

 Dianna knew she had a serious illness.

It wasn't just being overweight or obese any longer. Now she had something else, and she said, "I'm not just going to let this thing take me. I'm going to prepare to live well with or without this disease." It was bad. Sometimes, we couldn't even train. We would just have to stretch. Dianna, as I said previously, went through Steps One through Four. She didn't even realize she was doing the steps at the time. She was simply determined to do everything she could to feel better, look better, and have more energy.

 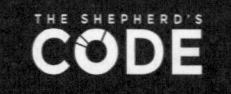

She's one of the most courageous women I know. She's amazing and determined. She wants to live; she doesn't want to die. And she wants to live well.

Step Six was hard for her because she would feel discouraged and depressed at times. She would be down and not want to exercise or do anything we were supposed to do together. I had to give her pep talks.

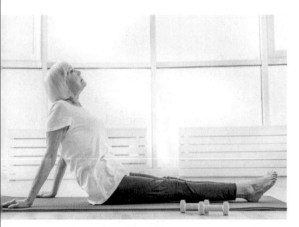

Dianna was one of those people with Parkinson's that you must make a conscious effort not to stare at. She was constantly moving like a noodle. Her body would do things that were out of control.

This shaking is called dyskinesia, which is a common symptom of Parkinson's. Some days, she was like a noodle, all over the place, and other days she was like a frozen statue. She would have no expression on her face, and she was very stiff. Even walking was a challenge. I never knew what to expect or what was going to come through the gym door.

My gym is a private studio for one-on-one clients and one-on-one training. Dianna and I did gait training, balance work, and all kinds of strength training. She lifted weights that were appropriate to help her with her functional movements like getting off the toilet, getting off the couch, getting out of a chair. You need muscle strength to perform those movements, but Parkinson's destroys the ability to move freely. All systems get attacked.

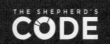

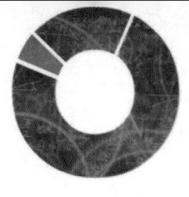
Believe it or not, because of Dianna's intelligence and determination, she had studied diets on her own. When I told her about *The Shepherd's Code System*, she said, "Oh, yeah. I've been doing some reading on different food plans, and I think that's the one that I like the most, the one with the low carbs, high fat and moderate protein." I said, "Well, that's it. That's huge, that's great," and she just got it.

 **She understood what to do.**

She was totally claiming it. There were times I would hand her two small balls, like two lacrosse balls, and I would say, "Juggle. I want to see you juggle." She would look at me like I was crazy, and I would say, "Look, studies show that juggling forces the brain to think a certain way and the body to respond a certain way. Juggling helps hand eye coordination. It is difficult for people without Parkinson's to juggle. It is even more difficult for people who have PD. Juggling stimulates the brain. It forces the brain to ask the body to do different motions at the same time. It's similar to playing the piano. The right hand and left hand are doing different movements at the same time. I need you to do this," and she would do it. She was willing to do pretty much anything I would throw at her, no pun intended, because sometimes I would throw a ball at her and see if she could catch it. Dianna was open to all my suggestions!

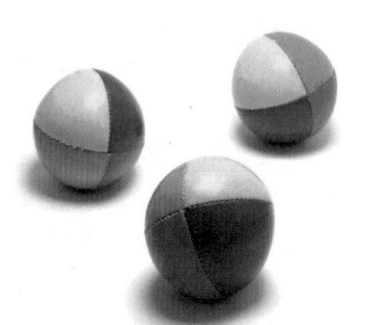

She had a deep trust in me, in *TSC*, in her training program, and in her abilities. She claimed it by doing all these things. I'll never forget the day she said, "I'm claiming this," which told me so much about her. Then, I knew she had the determination and the belief that this program was going to work. It's going to happen; it's going to be mine.

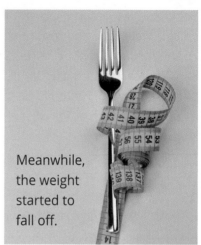

Meanwhile, the weight started to fall off.

She would come in each week, looking physically smaller.

She was excited about it, and she would tell me about new recipes she was trying, and how great her favorite snack was. Her physical shakes and erratic movements died down, and she became steadier with greater balance. She was able to focus more, and she continued to transform physically. She would tell me her weight every time she came in, "Guess what? I lost another five," or "I lost another three." Even when she plateaued with her weight loss, I would throw a suggestion out—a couple of high calorie days or intermittent fasting—and she immediately agreed, "Okay. What's that?" She was like a sponge. She just wanted to soak up everything I shared with her. She tried some of the things that help us get off a plateau and, sure enough, the weight continued to fall off. By following the steps and doing *TSC* and being so willing and believing that it was going to work, it did work—beautifully.

She lost a total of 60 pounds and, to this day, she's still losing weight. She has a goal weight in her mind, and she's not quite there, but almost.

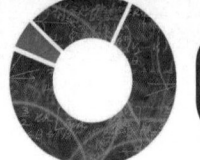
So, in about six months, Dianna lost 60 pounds. We still work together twice a week, and she continues to lose weight, and the beautiful thing is, she's losing fat not muscle. She'll always say to me, "Look at my bicep. You can see it now," and she'll flex. It's so cute and so awesome because now she has physical strength that she didn't have before, not even before she had Parkinson's.

🙂 She's stronger now, which is quite miraculous, and that strength helps her every day. Dianna has cut her work hours to part time. I'm glad that she has the financial ability to do that. She spends a lot of time at the gym, and she walks. If it's a nice day, she'll walk at the park with her husband. She does more physical things now because she can.

She's an inspiration because she had the world by the tail. She and her husband have a big house, their kids are grown and out of the house. They were getting ready for retirement and thinking about traveling around the world. Then Parkinson's hit. Dianna thought about giving up but quickly extinguished that thought and said to herself, "No, I'm not a quitter. I've never quit anything in my life, and I'm not going to start now." She continued to do her research, found me, and things have gotten better and better for her. For Dianna, resisting temptation meant resisting the desire to give up.

Dianna has Parkinson's disease, a very acute situation that she's had to accept. Many of you don't have a disease, thank goodness, but you may be overweight or you may feel awful and you want to feel better.

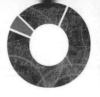

If you have Parkinson's, MS, ALS or any of those neurologically debilitating diseases, you too can "claim it,". You can claim dignity and a better life. You can feel energized if you set your mind to it and go through the steps just like Dianna did. But you don't need to be sick with a disease to be courageous and claim it like Dianna did. You can do it just the same way, even if you only want to feel better or lose some weight.

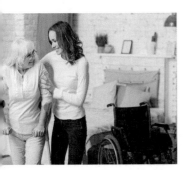

If Dianna can claim it while battling obesity, a lawyer's lifestyle and Parkinson's disease, you can, too. With *TSC*, you won't just lose weight, you develop much greater clarity of mind. The fog lifts, allowing you to be the best you can be.

I trained a gentleman named Don who also had Parkinson's, and he had a stroke (CVA) on top of Parkinson's. He came in, and at first I thought, "What the heck can I do with this person?" He cannot move his lower body, just the upper body from the waist up. We did a lot of upper body strengthening and stretching and all kinds of coordination exercises to help him, and he did amazingly well.

People were inspired by him; he affected people in the gym in a very positive way. He was another example of someone who was determined. He claimed it, tried *TSC System*, and had great success.

If you get started on *TSC* today, adopt the mindset, believe it's going to work, and claim it, you will absolutely decrease the chances of developing coronary artery disease, stroke, obesity, diabetes, and all the diseases related to being overweight. You can absolutely decrease your risk of disease and live a healthier, more dignified life.

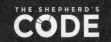

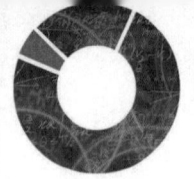

We're all going to die of something. Maybe it's old age, and that's fine. Eventually in old age, something gives out. We all have a ticket that will be punched some day; we just don't have the expiration date written down. We all have a choice to make. Do we want to take the steps necessary to increase our longevity in any way we can? Or are we going to say, "Oh, forget it. It's too hard," and not take steps to prevent certain things from happening?

We all want abounding energy; we want our hunger diminished so we're not always thinking about food; we want to sleep better; we would like to have increased mental focus.

By the time we are in our 30s, 40s and 50s, things in our bodies start to change. *TSC* helps keep things on track and keep you sharp.

Less dependence on medication means less money spent on medication for high blood pressure or high cholesterol. We want to be fat burners rather than sugar burners because it's healthier and it feels amazing!

> Most importantly, by claiming it with *TSC*, you will be more present. You'll begin to notice things, you'll be more aware in your life.

Even if you have a serious condition like Parkinson's or diabetes or Metabolic Syndrome, you can claim it. *The Shepherd's Code System* helps every kind of condition.

At least five times a week, I deal with people with MS or serious diabetes or Parkinson's. I had one client who was in her early 70's but highly functioning. She's had Parkinson's for ten years. She started *TSC* a few months ago, and already she said, "Kris, I have more energy than I've ever had in my life."

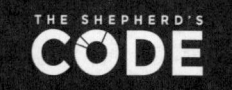

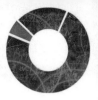

This may surprise you, but Alzheimer's and Parkinson's are similar in the way they work in the brain. In an uncontrolled clinical study published in the February 22nd, 2005 issue of the journal, Neurology, five patients followed a high-fat, low-carb, moderate-protein diet (which is what *TSC* is), for 28 days. Every single one of them, showed improvement in balance, tremors, shaking, and overall mood.

I work with all types of clients—some are young, some are old, some are overweight, some are underweight—all of them who have gone on *TSC* have seen amazing results. They have clarity, weight loss, increased energy and an overall zest for life that was lacking before *TSC*.

I work with a lot of women. These women in their 30's and 40's don't have a serious condition but have had a lot of difficulty finding a food plan that worked for them. When they went on *TSC*, they felt better physically, mentally and spiritually. They had all the wonderful results of glowing skin and feeling energized. To me, that's evidence that the *TSC System* is ideal for many people.

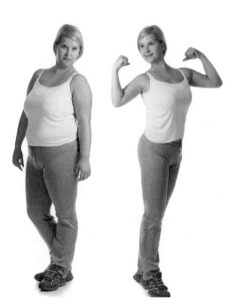

Some of my clients just do the exercise. They are still skeptical, and I try and not force it, because I don't want to do that. That doesn't work. I just tell them about it. I talk about it, and I say, "Look at me. I'm 52 years old, and I don't have a weight issue. I'm so lean, it's ridiculous, and I eat fat (lots of it) every day."

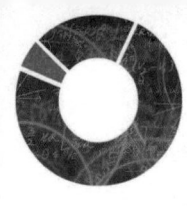
When most people think of diets, they think of restriction and deprivation and ugh, it's going to be horrible. With *TSC*, there's no deprivation. It's just the opposite.

I believe there is a plan for us, for every one of us, but if we are unable to tap into the desires of our heart, then we can't fulfill our purpose and be the best we can be; we miss out. We miss out on the job, the relationship or the opportunity presented.

A lot of people simply say, "It's okay to only have enough energy or enough will to just get through the day." But life can be so much more. One way to enjoy life more is to prepare for certain things. If you don't prepare, you can be blindsided by a disease, by an event, by anything that causes stress.

Change can be uncomfortable for most people. When you're not prepared, you are ill-equipped. If the doctor says, "Hey. You have diabetes, or you have high blood-sugar or guess what? Your blood pressure's too high," you're completely blindsided if you haven't mentally, physically, and spiritually prepared yourself.

What will your life look like if you do claim it? When you look ahead, you know good and bad things will happen. You know we're all going to get old and die; we might get a disease. But we can have a higher quality of life if we do certain things and claim it.

Are you going to have a high quality of life like Dianna? Are you going to claim it? If you do that, you can avoid a lot of potential problems! They don't have to be a part of your life.

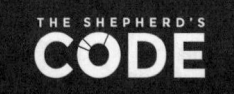

For example, if you decide to get up to get a drink out of the fridge, you don't sit and meditate and wonder whether you're actually able to so —you just get up out the the chair and go do what you intend, and don't think twice about it. Because you KNOW and you EXPECT and have no reason to DOUBT that you're going to do that thing. So you just do it. The same is with claiming our victory in *The Shepherd's Code*. Expect success!

If you claim it by using the *TSC System*, you will have all the wonderful benefits that it provides—the increased energy, the mental clarity and the obvious: weight loss. That will happen naturally. You will have less fat and much more muscle. Your risk for heart disease, diabetes, obesity, Alzheimer's, Parkinson's and seizures will decrease tremendously!

> **You'll also notice that your skin is clearer, and your stomach issues are much better.**

You'll also notice that your skin is clearer, and your stomach issues are much better. If you suffer from heartburn or IBS, they can be eliminated by using this food plan. When you are prepared and you're using *TSC*, if something were to happen like a cancer, you are in a place where you can do battle. You are much stronger, and you're able to fight. Your body can fight back.

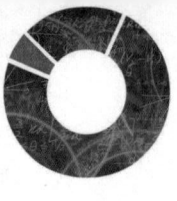

So many people I've seen in my years of being a trainer have suffered from different forms of cancer. The women I saw who were using *TSC* experienced a much better recovery. Not only was their recovery quicker, but they're still here today to talk about it. This is in stark contrast to some of the people I've met who had no interest in the diet or didn't believe that food could change their life.

Follow *The Shepherd's Code* and transform yourself. Claim it. In the next and final chapter of this book, we'll discuss Step Seven of *The Shepherd's Code*, "Maintain Your Strength and Dignity for a Lifetime."

 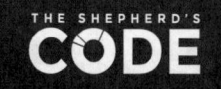

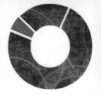

STEP 7: MAINTAIN YOUR STRENTH AND DIGNITY FOR A LIFETIME

One of my clients, Elaine, had brain cancer. When I met Elaine, she struck me as elegant. She had such a calming presence. She was a lovely lady and soft-spoken; when she spoke, people listened. She had that kind of effect on people. She was in her early 60's. She had two beautiful daughters, Nicole and Sunshine, and they too were my friends. I became friends with the whole family.

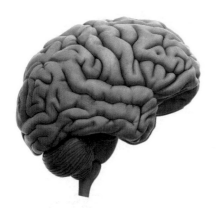

Elaine came to me because she said her doctors had told her she didn't have a lot of time, and that she needed to exercise because that would make her strong and help her maintain her dignity throughout the chemotherapy and surgeries.

I said, "Sure. Absolutely. Let's start working together." We did.

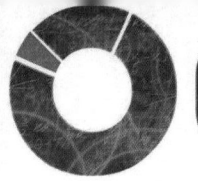
Elaine was following *The Shepherd's Code* without knowing it yet, which helped her brain function. She was extremely committed to doing whatever program I suggested. I suggested she come at least three times a week for thirty minutes. An hour was kind of hard for her because the brain cancer made her energy very low.

She asked me, "What about nutrition? Do you recommend anything, or is there some kind of diet that would help me have energy and function better?"

I said, "Actually, yes, I do."

I explained to her what *TSC* was and what foods she should be eating. I wrote up a little grocery list for her when her daughters took her to the supermarket. She said, "Wow! I kind of eat like this already. I might have a few sweets now and again." She said, "Kristina, if you're saying this is what I should do, I'm going to do it just the way you've written it down."

I said, "That's what I want to hear. That's awesome. Because if you really follow this the way it is written, your results will be quite positive.

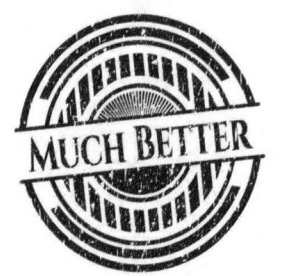

They'll be much closer to what you're looking for."

She began the *TSC System* when she started training with me, and she really liked it. She said it was easy. She said she felt better. She said, "I can't believe how clearly I can think." I said, "Isn't that a bonus?" Elaine was extremely enthusiastic about *TSC* and ended up being a very inspirational person in my own life.

I believe it took just a week for Elaine to start feeling positive results. Her daughters would call and text me me all the time about how she was doing and to thank me for helping their mom.

One of her daughters, Nicole, gave me a call and said, "Hey, I just want you to know Mom's doing great. She's doing much better, and she can't wait to tell you. She's so excited."

For a person who doesn't eat a lot of carbs, (for example, pasta, bread, or cereal every day), it's not difficult to transition into *TSC*. Elaine was not a big carb person or a sugar person, so it wasn't hard for her. She said, "Oh, I got a little tired the first day or two," but by the third day, she was doing great.

Elaine and I worked together consistently for six months. I promised that I would help her maintain her dignity at all costs. I told her, "I know this is important to you."

She was a beautiful woman. She was physically beautiful —tall, jet-black hair, and angular features. She was elegant-looking, and she was proud of her appearance because for her whole life, she'd been beautiful. I said, "You're not going to lose that. You will not lose your dignity or your self-respect. I promise you that. I will help you maintain that for as long as I possibly can. As long as you have breath in your body, you will have your dignity." She cried when she heard that. She cried and said, "Thank you."

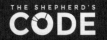

Elaine started training with me: exercise, balance, some gait training, some strength training, and some coordination training to help her with her daily activities. She would say to me, "Sometimes, I get dizzy. I have vertigo," which was a given because she had brain cancer.

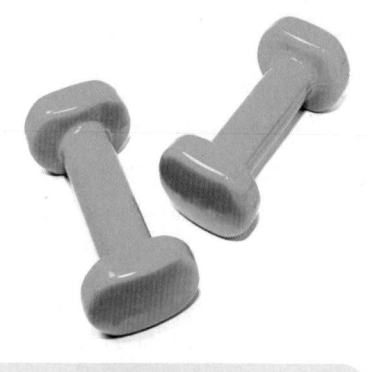

 **She had a huge inoperable tumor inside her head.**

We decided, she and I together, that we were going to work on the thing that bugged her the most, which was her balance. She would fall and trip, so we worked on fall prevention. I'd make her practice every single time we were together. I would put a flat mat on the floor with a fairly narrow ladder drawn on it. She would have to walk on it and not walk on the floor. I'd say, "Stay on the ladder. Can you do this?"

Then, I would put a little obstacle course in front of her, like a ball here or a shoe there. I would tell her, "Act like you're tripping. Pretend you don't see that," as if she were taking a walk outside. I showed her how to prevent falling, and she practiced. She got quite good at it as time passed.

TSC, in combination with what we were doing in the gym, helped her with her clarity, so she could hear what I was saying. She never said, "Wait, what? I don't understand. What are you talking about?" or "Do that again." She would say, "Okay," and get it the first time. Since Elaine had a brain tumor, the rest of her brain needed to function as well as possible. This food plan enabled her to do that.

One benefit of *The Shepherds Code* is the positive physical effects.

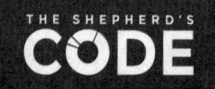

She became stronger. STRONGER TOGETHER

I put a ladder of kettlebells out, a 10-pound, a 20, a 30, and a 40, and she could deadlift every single one within a month or two of training with me, which is pretty impressive. I have people without a brain tumor that can't do that. As she continued the *TSC System*, she would come in smiling and bright and say, "Okay, let's go!" This was quite a contrast to when we first met. Then, her affect was flat. She didn't have a lot of energy, something she was craving, "I just want my energy back." As time went on, her energy improved. Her strength improved. Her mental clarity improved. It was awesome to watch.

Everything was going great. She was coming to me faithfully two or three times a week. We would do different things each time. She said, "You made this fun," and that meant the world to me.

One day about three weeks before she passed away, she came to the gym. I thought we were going to train, but she had a big bouquet of flowers. She was with her two daughters, and she came in and said, "Hi."

I said, "Hi. Why aren't you in your gym clothes?"

She said, "I'm done training for now. The doctor told me I have less than two weeks. I'm going to spend them with my daughters. They both took off work, and we're going to get our nails done and go to lunch and do all these fun things like see a play and go to movies." She was going to fill her days with her children and doing fun things, which I thought was great.

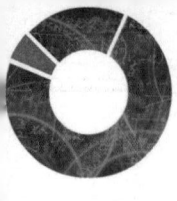

She gave me the flowers, and she thanked me for everything. Of course, I was crying, and she was crying, and pretty much everyone in the gym was crying. She said to me, "Kristina, Jesus never left me throughout this whole journey. He's never left me." That was profound, coming from a woman who was so close to death. She also said that faith is a gift, and all you must do is ask.

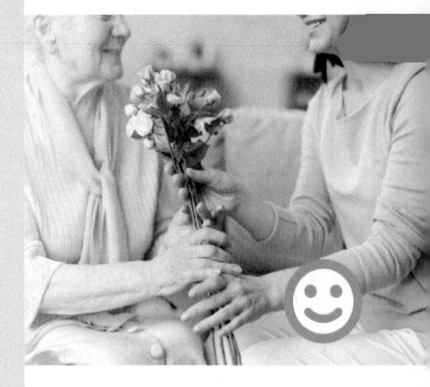

...and be content with what you have, for he has said, "I will never leave you nor forsake you."

Hebrews 13:5

I almost felt like I was listening to an angel when she was talking. I thought, "This is something huge that's happening right now." When I looked in her eyes, she still looked great. She said she felt great. She said, "I can't believe that I'm supposed to die in two or three weeks." She always maintained her sense of humor, which was kind of cool.

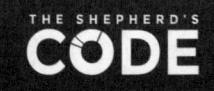

Her one daughter was in the medical field, so she was adept at this kind of thing and set hospice up for Elaine in her final weeks. The irony of this situation is that the two hospice nurses walked in and saw Elaine, Nicole, and Sunshine and said, "Okay, where's the patient? Where's the patient?" They all started laughing, giggling.

Elaine said, "That's me. That would be me."

The nurses were astounded at the way she looked. They couldn't believe that she was walking, talking, and getting up off the sofa by herself. They said, "Well, are you sure? Are you sure we're supposed to...? Are we in the right house?" Elaine got a big kick out of that.

Elaine's daughter, Nicole, called me about a week after she came to the gym with the flowers. She said, "Kris, if you want to see Mom and talk to her, you should come now."

I said, "Sure. Absolutely."

Elaine only lived five minutes from me. I went to her house. I thought, "I'm not going to cry. I'm not going to act all sad. I'm going to be happy, make her laugh, and we'll have a nice time." So, that's what I did. I went to her house. She was sitting in her favorite chair, covered in her favorite blanket, and we just talked. She said, "I really like your outfit." and I said, "Well, I like yours too."

Then we just kind of laughed, and she again thanked me. She just couldn't say enough about how much she appreciated having her dignity. She said, "Kristina, I'll never forget those words, and you were true to your promise," she said.

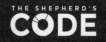

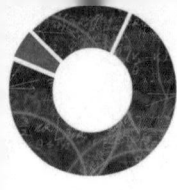
I said, "Well, you did a really good job, too, Elaine. You worked hard, and that's a credit to you." She was so courageous... so courageous.

Her daughters were there, and we had a nice conversation. When I left, of course, I was bawling. So were her girls. I gave her a big hug, and I said, "I will see you on the other side."

After my last visit with Elaine, I kept texting her daughters, "How are you doing? Everything okay? Well—Did it happen?"

They would say, "Nope. Mom's doing fine."

She passed away two weeks later, which blew the doctors away because she was supposed to have died a month or two before that.

She did pass away at night in her bed, and it was very peaceful. I received a call from her daughters saying, "We're going to have a memorial service here at the house on Saturday. We would love for you to be there."

I said, "Of course I'll be there," so I went that Saturday to the memorial service.

They had pictures of Elaine with me and with the woman, Amy, who owns the studio. There was a picture of Elaine and me exercising, and she seemed so happy. There were pictures of her throughout her lifetime. I thought, "What an incredible woman she was; remarkable—her spirit and her faith and her tenacity to not give up."

 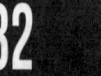

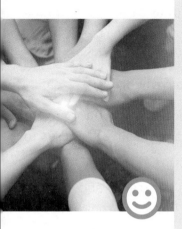

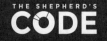

TSC and any exercise that went with it assured that to the end of her life she could remain strong and dignified. She maintained her glow, even though they had her on steroids and all kinds of things. She still looked beautiful. *TSC* helped with that. It also helped maintain her strength and her mental clarity. It kept her from falling apart. Especially when it was combined with the exercise routine.

TSC MENTALITY FOR LIFE

I know that you, like Elaine, want to maintain your strength, your health, and your dignity for as long as possible, but you feel terrible because you haven't started a eating plan that works or you haven't begun to exercise or do things that you feel you should. The *TSC System* will be a very good beginning to restoring strength, health, and dignity for a lifetime.

Bill Wilson, who was the founder of Alcoholics Anonymous, said, "I am most impressed with the ability of a high-fat, low-carb diet to improve brain function. This is not just true for those with obvious brain disorders. It also applies to those who are quite healthy. In this complex world, full of daily stresses, getting a leg up when it comes to brain function can improve your life in a multitude of ways. On the other hand, if you want to guarantee declining brain function, I suggest sticking to the standard American diet."

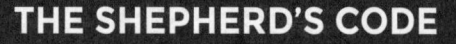
I agree with Mr. Wilson, 100%. The standard American diet is lacking in so many ways. It's filled with processed foods and carbs, and not the good carbs, either. It advocates, "Oh, you must eat three meals a day." Really? Well, who said that? I don't. I believe that's a heap of lies.

Low fat, low sugar, three squares whether you're hungry or not, eat.

That's not really what our bodies want to do. They don't want to eat necessarily three times a day or four times a day. You're supposed to eat when you're hungry.

If a woman with brain cancer can maintain her dignity and strength through *TSC*, anyone can. She had faith. She had very strong faith, and I hope that her story inspires you.

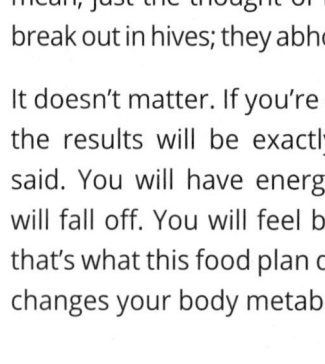

Elaine exercised throughout her six months with me. She exercised, and she did the *TSC System*. It was great. It was a wonderful combination that helped her maintain her strength throughout her journey, but I've met many people, even some of my clients, who hate exercise. I mean, just the thought of it makes them break out in hives; they abhor it that much.

It doesn't matter. If you're following TSC, the results will be exactly as we have said. You will have energy. The weight will fall off. You will feel better because that's what this food plan does for you. It changes your body metabolically.

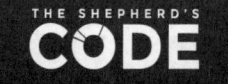

But exercise does help. If you want to see results much more quickly, exercise can be key. But again, if you don't like it or you don't have time, it is not necessary.

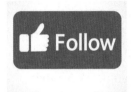

I promise you, the same way I promised Elaine—If you follow *TSC*, you will have dignity and strength throughout your lifetime. If you trust me and follow *TSC* as described in this book, you will—this is a promise—you will have results which include increased energy, weight loss, and health.

If you don't decide to try *TSC* and you continue to maintain whatever food plan or lack of a food plan that you have, you can expect more of the same— more of the same issues, more of the same problems, more of the same illnesses.

The Shepherd's Code is wonderful not only for preventing certain things from developing, but also for nipping things in the bud once you've already developed a condition. It's part of your arsenal of things to keep you well, to keep you protected, and to keep you healthy. If you choose to take that armor off, you'll chose to be vulnerable.

Some people tell me, "Well, my grandpa lived until a ripe old age of 99 years old. He smoked, and he drank, and he partied, and he didn't have any health problems. He had fun while he was here."

Well, that's great, but how many of those cases really exist? How many of those grandpas are there who can do all those things and not have an issue? I believe there are very few. Risks like that are like taking your life, throwing the dice and saying, "Hey. I'm going to live this way. I'm going to continue to smoke, drink, party, eat cake, and eat cookies, and we'll see what happens."

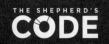

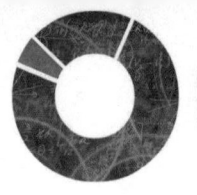

CONCLUSION

The trade-off? Vitality, energy, a zest for life and maintaining your strength and dignity for a lifetime. Boom. Period. There is one obvious choice, *The Shepherd's Code System*.

The studies, testimonies and my experience tell volumes of what it can do for you! I have blessed to have been able to share *TSC* with Elaine and all my clients. Those who jump on board have amazing results. Those that choose not to, will never know.

I hope you are one of those who choose to jump aboard! It's a wonderful ride.

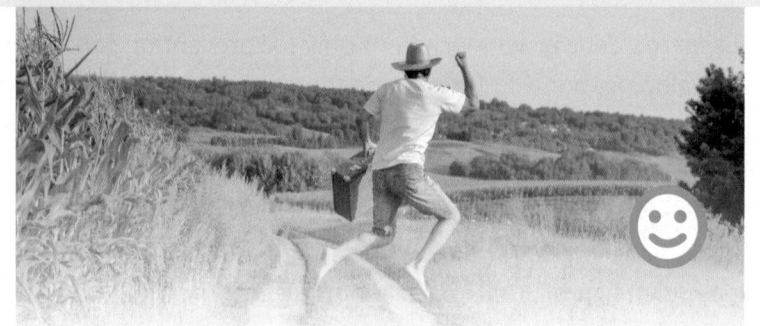

I went to an endocrinologist last week who specializes in hormone therapy. She has a machine reads your body fat, body weight, your BMI and your basal metabolic rate (the calories you burn if you just were lying in bed doing absolutely nothing). It also tells your muscle mass versus your skeletal mass and how much water is in your body. I believe this machine is used by the NFL. It's very accurate. Football players and professional athletes love this because it helps them tell where they are in their progress for their goals.

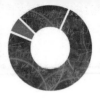

I got on the machine, and was so excited to see that even now, when I'm really at a level of excellent weight, body fat and muscle mass, my body fat is still decreasing. I burned another 2%, and my muscle mass went up by six pounds!

Some women would be upset, "Oh my gosh. This is crazy. I gained six pounds." But when you look at what this machine is telling you regarding body fat versus muscle mass, who cares what you weigh if you have 16% body fat and are female? For a woman that's pretty low; it's considered athlete level.

> This was more evidence of *TSC* at work and how it truly, truly changes lives.

That's how *TSC* continues to work miracles in my life. I've demonstrated throughout this book how it does the same and more for all kinds of people, and I see the results daily in my work as a trainer and nutritionist.

We've discussed a woman with brain cancer, a woman with Parkinson's, and the average housewife just trying to feel better, do a good job and look good. We've looked at a woman who is in recovery from alcoholism, and a young girl in her mid-20s. We've also discussed my client Brad who has seen miraculous results.

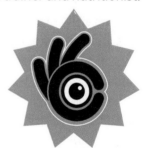

TSC works wonders with so many different types of people. It can help you if you're chronically overweight, tired, sick, and/or frustrated because you can't find a diet that will help you lose weight and improve your overall health and fitness.

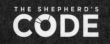

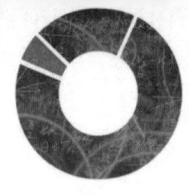
And it can work even if you doubt whether you have the time, self-discipline, or desire to commit to a new lifestyle, or whether you worry about having enough money to buy healthy food. It will help you if you feel guilty or uncomfortable about making an investment of time and money in your diet and health, or you don't think you can resist the temptations of food and drink, or family and friends who aren't on the same program.

> This incredible, fat-burning food plan, this diet of "healing fats", is for anyone at any age, no matter how healthy or unhealthy they are right now. Quite simply, it's the best way to eat, stay healthy and strong and to look your best for a lifetime.

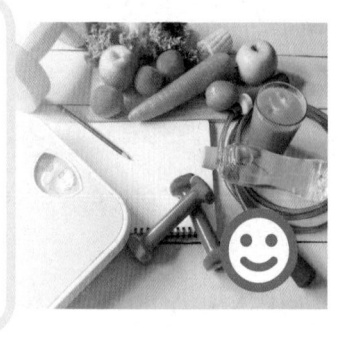

I work with a wide variety of people in my practice. I'm working with a young guy who's about 38 years old right now. He doesn't have a serious illness like some of my clients, but he really wanted to improve his overall health and fitness, and he has. We're making progress every day, but he's already dropped his body fat by 5% and increased his weight by seven pounds. Even though he's gained weight, he's gotten smaller. His jeans were falling from his waist, and his shirtsleeves became tight from his muscles. He was so excited. His name is David, and he still trains with me. He's a perfect example of a guy with no illness who just wanted to get bigger, look better, and have more energy. He tried everything, eating a lot of carbs thinking that would help him with his muscle gain, but it didn't.

As you know by now, I discovered the *TSC System* through a combination of trial-and-error, serendipity, and divine intervention. I have over

 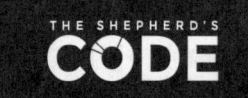

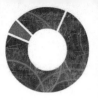
20 years' experience working with overweight people, underweight people, people who want to compete in bodybuilding, people that want to tone and not build a lot of muscle, and those who want to look firmer and be stronger. I've worked with kids, teenagers, all kinds of people from all walks of life.

I was also married to someone who had a fatal disease called ALS, and was his primary caregiver. Throughout that journey, I learned a lot about food, what's healthy, what's not, what would be the best for his brain function during his time here, and what would help his quality of life the most. I researched everything about food plans and exercise. Everything that we could control, I researched.

I've earned different certifications in health, fitness, and nutrition throughout my lifetime as my interests changed, and I've become more aware of what works and doesn't work. Crossfit was supposed to be great because it helped with functional movement, so I got certified in crossfit. Then, I was asked to head up a kids' program at my gym, so I got certified in Crossfit for kids. My dad used to call me "the perpetual student." He said, "You'll always be in school for something." I think that was a compliment.

After doing Crossfit for over five years, I thought, "You know, this is great. It's not a bad thing, but for people who are sick, or women who really don't want to lift heavy stuff, you have to moderate it and scale it down." I went back for HIIT training. That's high intensity interval training. I use that, or Tabata, which really burns fat and stokes your metabolism.

I have all this experience with many different types of programs that are successful and help people reach their goals.

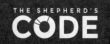

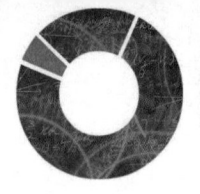

Mothers are often told, "Oh, kids need fat. Feed them whole milk and peanut butter and other high-fat food." When I had my son Luke, I thought it would be important to know if that were true. It's true. I got certified as a child obesity specialist, just to make sure I knew everything I could about nutrition for small children and babies. Today, I still work as a trainer for a diverse population. It's my passion and my goal to help people with their fitness and health to help them reach their full potential.

Throughout my lifetime and journey to the place where I am today, I have suffered with bulimia and anorexia. I had an issue with drinking too much alcohol at one point in my life.

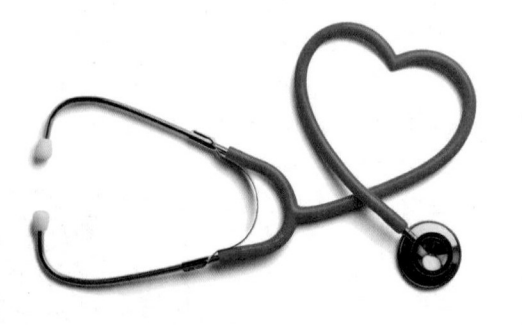

I've experienced a lot of challenging times. I understand so well how food is a drug and how sugar especially can just wreak havoc within your body, your mind and your life, especially when all you do is think about it.

You're obsessed with sugar because it feels so good when you initially put it in your mouth. Of course, you then feel horrible later, and the guilt just perpetuates the cycle. You feel guilty, so then you eat more to feel better. So then you feel worse, and it goes on and on until somehow, someway you break that cycle.

When I went to rehab as a young woman, the seed was planted regarding a relationship with Jesus. Truths started to become clear and I understood which direction was right.

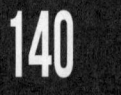
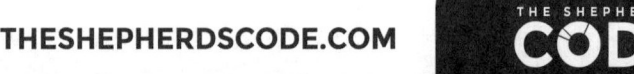

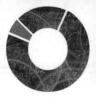

I learned that everything we do in our lives is related to our health: what we're thinking, what we're eating, what we're doing. It all relates to our health and well-being. When this seed was planted, it opened up a whole world of hope for me.

Rehab was the garden where the seed was first planted. I watered it, and it grew into something beautiful.

I kept researching and trying different things with my food plan. I learned that when I ate carbs, even though experts said they were okay to eat (carbs like potatoes, bananas, and beans), I didn't feel well. I didn't feel lean. I felt bloated and tired. Maybe I'd get a headache. Different symptoms from different foods were happening, and I decided to eliminate them. That's how I came to realize that increasing fat and decreasing carbs was the ideal balance for me and for lots of others.

Through experimentation and trial and error with different foods I discovered that some really are "healing fats". I found this in rehab over 20 years ago, then through scientific journals. *TSC* recommends specifically what fats to eat and I support that.

I wrote this book to introduce you to the *TSC System*. It's a step-by-step weight loss program that works by eating more fat ("healing fats") and fewer carbs. Scientific evidence supports the benefits of this plan. I think this is what makes *TSC* so different and so amazingly successful. It is a low-carb, high-fat, moderate-protein food plan that works.

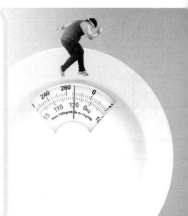

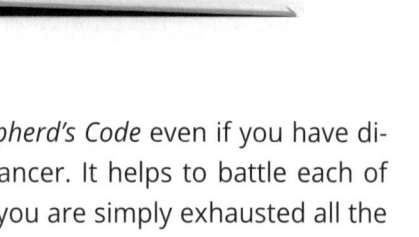
When you follow the recommendations in this book, you will gain the results that we talked about, the high energy and the weight loss. At the same time, you are protecting yourself from disease in later life.

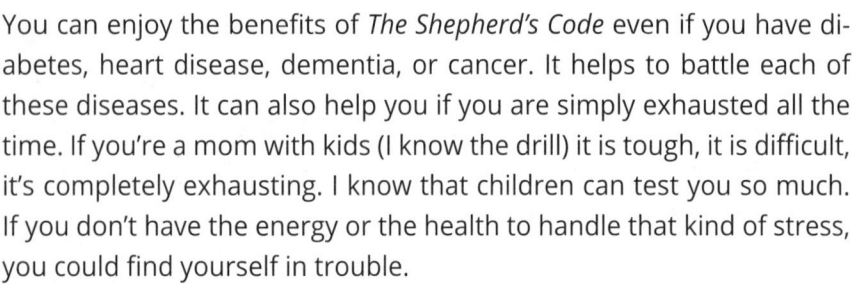

You can enjoy the benefits of *The Shepherd's Code* even if you have diabetes, heart disease, dementia, or cancer. It helps to battle each of these diseases. It can also help you if you are simply exhausted all the time. If you're a mom with kids (I know the drill) it is tough, it is difficult, it's completely exhausting. I know that children can test you so much. If you don't have the energy or the health to handle that kind of stress, you could find yourself in trouble.

TSC also helps with weight loss, of course. That's the obvious. It helps with food addiction. If you're battling some type of food addiction or addiction to sugar, this diet is very beneficial.

TSC is not expensive. You don't have to buy ingredients to make fancy meals. You don't need tons of money or a personal chef to do it the way we suggest in this book. It is simple; it's straightforward and user friendly. It's easy—easy to understand.

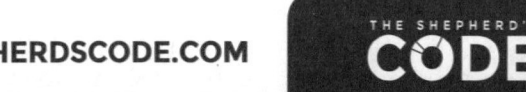

If you decide to exercise while doing *TSC*, your results will come more quickly, but you do not have to exercise when you do this diet.

My sister was a perfect example. She didn't exercise one minute and lost 12 pounds in a period of two weeks.

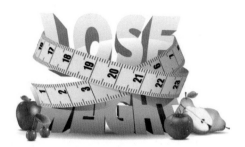

Just follow the seven steps outlined in this book and start your journey to freedom, health and wellness.

1. Develop the TSC mindset.
2. Free yourself from food addiction.
3. Get started on the ideal you.
4. Rest and eat right.
5. Resist temptation.
6. Claim it.
7. Maintain your strength and dignity for a lifetime.

Someone said to me once, "Kristina, are you sick and tired of being sick and tired?" When they asked me that question, it was like a light bulb went off in my mind, and I thought, "Yes, I am sick and tired of being sick and tired."

I couldn't do all the things I wanted to or enjoy life like I wanted to, so I decided to make a change. If you're ready to make a change, trust me

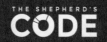

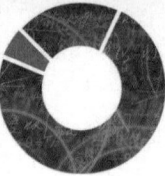

and take these seven steps. Take the steps, do *TSC*, and you can absolutely, positively expect right-off-the-bat weight loss. That's the initial benefit, not to mention the mental clarity. You'll be astounded by the way you can think, and your energy will be through the roof.

This is not just a diet; it's a lifestyle. It's a way to change your life to be the best you can be.

Along with the physical benefits of utilizing the *TSC System*, there are also the spiritual benefits that we talked about. You will be so fully present in your life, abundant in energy, awareness and focus. You won't be numb or in a brain fog.

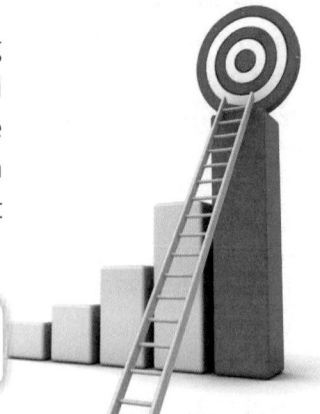

The choice is yours.

I have explained to you the seven steps to take with *TSC*. I have talked to you about my sister and other people that I've worked with who have had a lot of success with this diet.

I've given you some scientific background about why it works and how it works.

We have talked about the different diseases like diabetes, chronic fatigue, coronary artery disease, obesity, depression, and even low self-esteem that the diet combats.

We have discussed different menu plans; I've given you examples and shakes that are wonderful, especially if you're under stress.

We've also talked about being on vacation or having a lifestyle that includes eating out regularly. It is very possible and easy to stay on *TSC*.

I've given you a grocery list and some sample meals.

 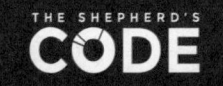

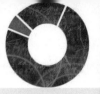

THE SHEPHERD'S CODE

It's simple and straightforward. There's no trick. There's no, "When is the other shoe going to drop?" There's no catch. There's no gimmick. This is really what it is. It is a food plan/lifestyle that will keep you forever in the best shape, in the best mind frame, and in the best spiritual condition that you can imagine. It covers all the areas of life.

Now, it's up to you. You do have a choice. You can stay with what you're doing in your so-called comfort zone, or you can step out of it and create the new you. You've got nothing to lose, nothing at all except weight.

"By faith Abraham obeyed when he was called to go out to a place that he was to receive as an inheritance. And he went out, not knowing where he was going."

Hebrews 11:8

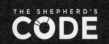

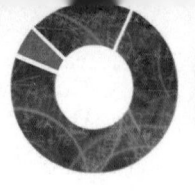
I will be there along the way to help and guide you on your journey. You can contact me; I can be your coach. What other diet has that? I am a person who has been where you are. I've experienced the food addiction, the bulimia, the depression, the death of a loved one, all of that. I am your go-to person. If you're not sure of what decision to make or the results aren't happening as quickly as you would like, it's always nice to have someone to reach out to who can help you stay on your path.

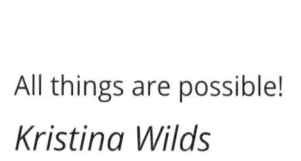

And if you purchased this book but haven't joined our community and would like more information on how you can transform yourself and gain back your energy and youthful appearance, go to **shepcode.com/members**. I hope you too will join the tens of thousands that have achieved success following *The Shepherds Code*.

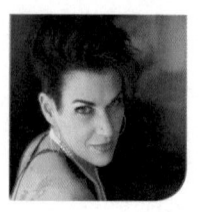

All things are possible!

Kristina Wilds

72-HOUR QUICK START GUIDE

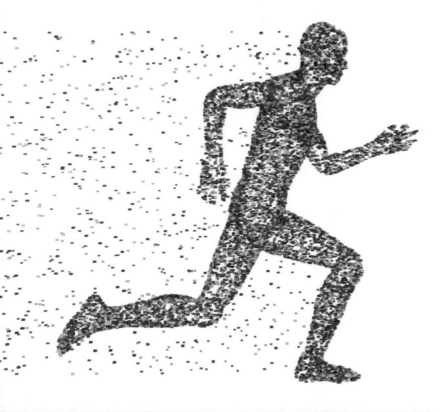

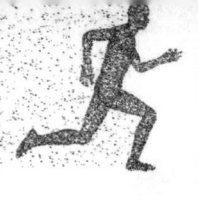

THE SHEPHERD'S
CODE

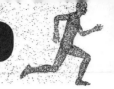

The contents of this document are based upon my opinions of *The Shepherd's Code* unless otherwise noted. This work is intended to share knowledge and information learned through research, experience, and discussions with others. The opinions of others, such as in the comments and the forum, are their own and are not endorsed by *The Shepherd's Code*. The information contained herein is not intended to diagnose, treat, cure or prevent any condition or disease, but rather to provide general information that is intended to be used for educational purposes only. Please consult with your physician or healthcare practitioner if you have any concerns. By using, viewing and interacting with *The Shepherd's Code* or **shepherdscode.com** website, you agree to all terms of engagement, thus assuming complete responsibility for your own actions. The authors and publishers will not claim accountability, nor shall they be held liable for any loss or injury sustained by you. Use, view and interact with these resources at your own risk. All products and information given to you by *The Shepherd's Code* and its related companies are strictly for informational purposes only. While every attempt has been made to verify the accuracy of information provided on our website and within our publications, neither the authors nor the publishers are responsible for assuming liability for possible inaccuracies. The authors and publishers disclaim any responsibility for the inaccuracy of the content, including but not limited to errors or omissions. Loss of property, injury to self or others, and even death could occur as a direct or indirect consequence of the use and application of any content found herein. Please act responsibly. The information provided may need to be downloaded and/or viewed using third party software, such as Acrobat. It's the user's responsibility to install the software necessary to view such information. Any downloads, whether purchased or given for free from our website, related websites or hosting systems are performed at the user's own risk. Although we take great preventative measures, we cannot warranty that our websites are free of corrupting computer codes, viruses or worms. If you are a minor, you can use this service only with permission and guidance from your parents or guardians.

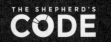

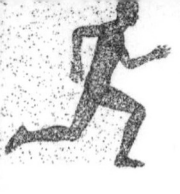

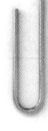

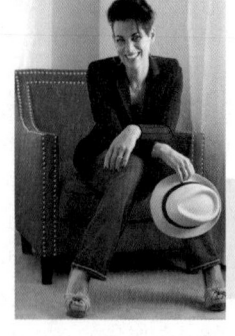

Hi, It's Kristina here... Congratulations and WELCOME to *The Shepherd's Code Family!*

I'm delighted you have chosen to **join this like-minded community.**

Your choice to join this community is going to change your life for the better in more ways than you would probably **believe.**

Here's what a few of our members say about *The Shepherd's Code System:*

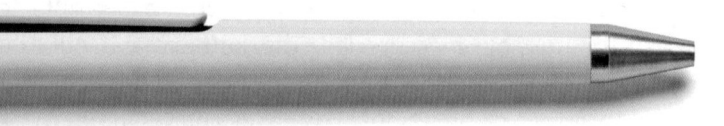

Monica K.
37 years old

I began *The Shepherd's Code* and my belly fat is diminishing before my eyes!! I feel energetic and happy. My mood is so much better every day. My coworkers keep asking, 'what are you doing…?'

 32   42 Comments

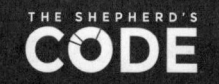

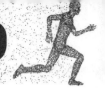

Mackenzie C.
20 years old

I was so conditioned to believe that fat was bad, it was hard for me to believe this would help me lose weight! However, when I looked at Kristina (52 years old), I couldn't believe this woman (old enough to be my mom) was so full of energy, lean and really strong! I had to try *TSC*. I have continued to lose weight and am down another 20lbs since I started…

 28

12 Comments

Kim P.
48 years young

I started *The Shepherd's Code System* right away! Within three days, people started commenting on my appearance. They said something looked different but really good. Within two weeks, I had lost 12lbs.!! I didn't exercise, calorie count or weigh and measure! I ate until I was satiated and that was it! I feel so amazing today.

 26

9 Comments

Amy M.
27 year old

My muscle to fat ratio has changed dramatically. My body fat is down and my muscle mass is up! I am so excited to see where I will be in a few more months from now! I am grateful for Kristina and her encouragement, support and empathy!

 32

13 Comments

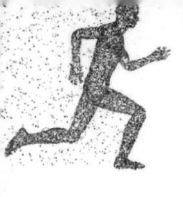
 Mary O.
72 years young

I found the system so simple to follow. My energy is up and I have dropped two dress sizes! I love the ease of *TSC* and how I am rarely hungry. Parkinson's Disease saps energy and *TSC* helps replace it…!

👍 32

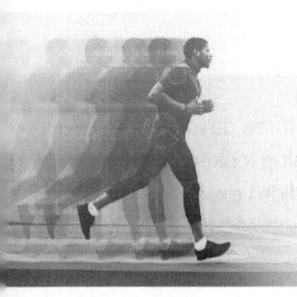

In just a few days of following *The Shepherd's Code*, you'll notice changes in your body, mind and in your spirit… and in just a couple of weeks you'll not only look more fit, but will also be bursting with energy you forgot was even possible.

And that's why I want to congratulate you on your choice to start this journey. Together, and with the guidance of the Holy Spirit, we will find our fullness in a healthy life driven by the purposes and wholeness He has set out of us.

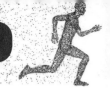

IMAGINE YOURSELF A COUPLE OF WEEKS FROM NOW:

Weight Loss: Kicking the sugar habit and turning your body into a healing, fat-melting machine will make you leaner and lighter, with no bloating or tummy issues.

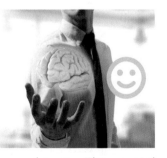

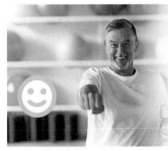

Increased Energy: *The Shepherd's Code* will make you feel like you're on a drug that gives you extra energy throughout the day, but it's just your food plan maximizing your biology the way nature intended. You will be able to use your talents more effectively and efficiently!

Greater Clarity and Mental Focus: By improving brain health and mitochondrial energy, *The Shepherd's Code* will have you laser-focused on what matters most to you each day. It's a priceless gift that can help you in all aspects of your life by allowing you to be more present with family, friends,

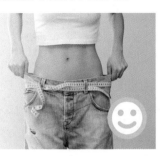

co-workers, community, and of course, your soul mate. The mental clarity on this diet, which you begin to feel in about four or five days, is amazing. You will find more connectedness in prayer, wisdom from what you learn, and clarity to make righteous decisions about your life.

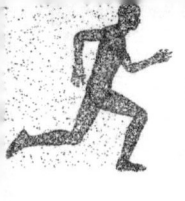
Enhanced Athletic Performance and Endurance: There's nothing

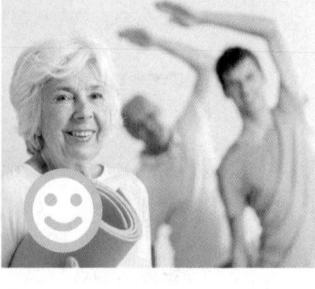

like a stable, constant source of energy to enhance your athletic performance and endurance, and that's what *The Shepherd's Code* will give you. You will be able to execute your God given roles with excellence and vigor.

Disease Prevention and Mitigation: Studies and my own experience demonstrate that *The Shepherd's Code* can help you prevent, reduce, or mitigate the effects of certain diseases

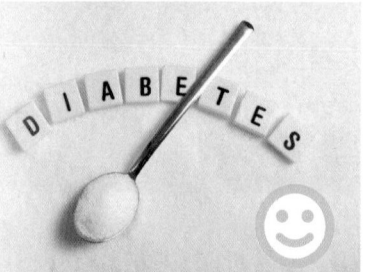

and ailments, such as type 2 diabetes, Parkinson's, Alzheimer's, epilepsy, and coronary artery disease. It mitigates or eliminates candida by not feeding it. (Candida is yeast, and it lives off unhealthy, sugary carbs, which are not included in *The Shepherd's Code*). And *The Shepherd's Code* starves cancer cells. Cancer hates ketones, and that's what *The Shepherd's Code* produces in your body. Pretty good deal, wouldn't you say?

Alleviation of Acne and Other Skin Problems: *The Shepherd's Code* often alleviates or eliminates acne, rosacea, eczema, psoriasis, and

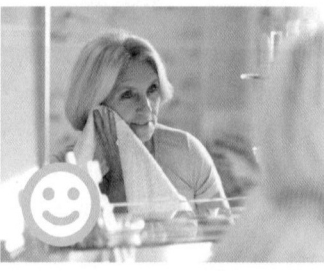

even dandruff. I had a 20-year-old client who was very pretty but plagued with some skin issues, for example. She had acne and a little bit of rosacea, and she tried everything.

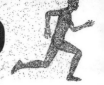

So I said, "Hey, why don't you try *The Shepherd's Code*? It's a wonderful system, and it really helps to clear up acne or any kind of skin issue." Well, within a week she noticed a difference, and within two weeks her face was radiant. It was beautiful. She was thrilled.

Acid Reflux Relief: In many cases *The Shepherd's Code* drastically reduces acid reflux, and I can attest to this from personal experience because I used to have heartburn all the time before I discovered *TSC*. I know so many people who complain of heartburn, and, "Oh, my esophagus. You know, I feel like it's always stuck. Nothing ever helps. It's always on 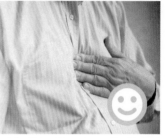 fire." They need to stop complaining and try *The Shepherd's Code*. You'll enjoy the blessing of your food rather than dread the aftereffects.

Improved Fertility: Studies on women trying to get pregnant show that *TSC System* improves fertility as well. Women on high fat, low carb, moderate protein diets like *The Shepherd's Code* were able to conceive much more quickly than those who weren't. Perhaps you will "fill your quiver" much more easily than you had expected!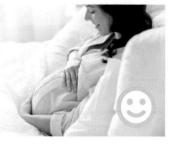

> *Behold, children are a heritage from the Lord, the fruit of the womb a reward. Like arrows in the hand of a warrior are the children of one's youth. Blessed is the man who fills his quiver with them!*
>
> **Psalm 127:3-5**

In fact, your friends and family will be telling you how much of a difference they can see in no time at all...

They will compliment your looks and your energy... and they will want to know your secret...

HOW TO USE
THE SHEPHERD'S CODE:

1. Visit **www.shepcode.com/members**
2. Simply enter the same email address you signed up with (there are no passwords).
3. Join our *TSC Family Facebook Group* for continued support and great recipes by going to **www.shepcodefamily.com**

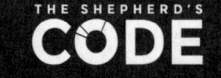

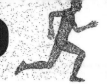

As soon as you login to the membership site, you can click on the images to download your full *The Shepherd's Code System.*

To get started immediately, download and print out the **WWJE Grocery Field Guide** and take it to the grocery store with you. Once you have filled your shopping cart with all these fresh, organic and omega-3 rich "healing fats", you'll be able to create nearly unlimited delicious recipes.

The Shepherd's Code System is EASY – all you need to remember is: High Fat, Moderate Protein, and Low Carbohydrates in your diet that will look like this – **75/20/5** fats being the highest and carbs being the lowest! If you eat with this combination and keep your daily carbohydrate intake below 20 grams you are **GUARANTEED** to turn your body into a **fat-melting machine** in as little as 3 days... and all without stepping foot in the gym!

IMPORTANT: When counting carbs make sure to subtract the fiber from the total carbs since your body will not digest those. Also, sometimes you will see "sugar alcohols" on labels. You can subtract those carbs from the total as well.

> *I appeal to you therefore, brothers, by the mercies of God, to present your bodies as a living sacrifice, holy and acceptable to God, which is your spiritual worship.*
>
> **Romans 12:1**

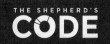

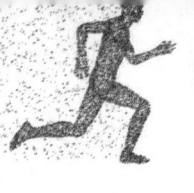
To get to the place where our bodies are a living sacrifice, we need to be rid of the things that we allow to control our minds, behaviors, and priorities. We hardly realise it, but with a daily regimen that includes eating so frequently, we sometimes let even thoughts of food push God out of his proper position of being first in our lives. When even food becomes an obsession, it is time for an overhaul.

Before we get to the 3-Day *The Shepherd's Code* Meal Plan there's something important for you to realize. There is a very good chance your body is addicted to sugar (by living off a consistent diet high in carbs).

BUT I WANT TO KNOW HOW MUCH I SHOULD EAT!

Then follow these 3 simple rules:

FAT:
as much as you want

PROTEIN:
half your weight in grams of protein
Example:
200LBS / 2 = 100G of protein per day

CARBS:
eat less than 20g per day

5%
20%
75%

- Fats
- Protein
- Carbs

 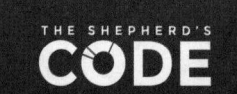

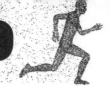

There will be a detox period where you might feel some flu like symptoms, which are very common when your body transitions from burning sugar as its main fuel source to burning fat. The good news is you can help alleviate the symptoms if you follow these guidelines:

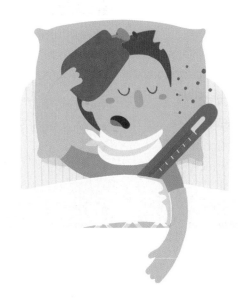

GET OVER THE
KETO FLU

What is Keto Flu?

In order for your body to flip the Master Metabolic Switch from burning glucose to burning fat you'll go through a short 2-4 day transition period where you might have flu like symptoms. It's a completely normal detox known as keto flu. Don't worry, there are simple solutions for this as you'll see here.

Keto Flu Symptoms:

- Muscle cramps
- Skin problem
- Nausea
- Lightheadedness
- Constipation
- Fatigue
- Headache
- Hypertension
- Brain fog
- Drowsiness

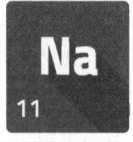

Mg
12

Magnesium

You need: 300 mg/day
You will need more if you are active.

Sources:
- Artichoke
- Spinach
- Fish
- Dark chocolate
- Nuts

Deficiency:
- Muscle cramps
- Irritable
- Dizziness
- Fatigue

K
19

Potassium

You need:
1000 mg/day

Sources:
- Mushrooms
- Avocado
- Salmon
- Dark chocolate
- Nuts

Deficiency:
- Abdominal cramps
- Constipation
- Weakness
- Nausea
- Hypertension

Na
11

Sodium

You need: 5000 mg/day
From natural food

Sources:
- Bacon
- Salt
- Fish
- Bouillon/broth
- Spinach

Deficiency:
- Nausea
- Muscle cramps
- Confusion
- Headache
- Fatigue

Keto tip

Embrace "healing fats." That's right, eat lots of grass fed fatty meat, bacon, butter, coconut oil and even heavy cream in your coffee. Make sure you are consuming 75% fats in your daily diet. That is what will turn your body into a fat melting machine.

Keto tip

Be careful not to consume too much protein. Excess protein in your body can turn into glucose. You want to limit yourself to 20% proteins per day. So get over your fear of fats making you fat and embrace "healing fats" and watch the pounds melt away.

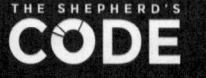

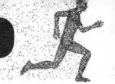

THE SHEPHERD'S CODE
72-HOUR QUICK-START MEAL PLAN

The Shepherd's Code book has all the information you need as well as the 7-step system to lose weight, look great, and feel younger.

However, many *TSC* clients are excited to get started immediately. That's why I created this 3-day quick start guide.

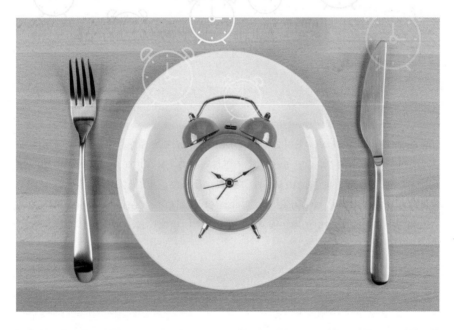

I started using this many moons ago, first with myself and then with all of my clients. After the three days, you will feel so great you will want to keep going, so consider this a jump-start. I've created **a delicious three-day meal plan** to turn your body into a fat-melting machine.

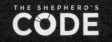

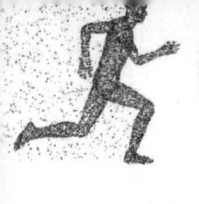

> *Blessed be the God and Father of our Lord Jesus Christ! According to his great mercy, he has caused us to be born again to a living hope through the resurrection of Jesus Christ from the dead*
>
> **1 Peter 1:3**

It's exciting when we realize that being born again is just the start of a whole new life where everything is seen through a different set of lenses. In much the same way *The Shepherd's Code System* allows you a fresh start that will provide a straighter path, a cleaner way of life, and healing that you never knew was at your fingertips.

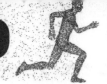

DAY ONE

Breakfast:
- Cream Cheese Pancakes with butter and sugar free syrup (if desired)
- coffee with heavy cream (& no-carb sweetener if desired)
- bacon or sugar free breakfast sausage

What are Cream Cheese Pancakes? Simply take a cup of cream cheese and 2 or 3 eggs add a dash of vanilla and blend in a blender! Cook in a pan just like regular pancakes. Be sure to use butter for your pan and on your pancakes before serving. Delicious!!
TIP: To make the pancakes fluffier and easier to work with, add another half cup of cream cheese and 1/8 tsp of baking powder.

Snack: 2 or 3 sticks of string cheese or handful of salted almonds

Lunch:
Ham and cheese rolled with mayonnaise and arugula or spinach... and feel free to replace mayonnaise with cream cheese if you prefer.

Snack: Half an avocado with lite salt and pepper

Dinner:
- Buffalo chicken wings, grilled
- Sugar-free blue cheese dressing
- Celery sticks

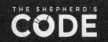

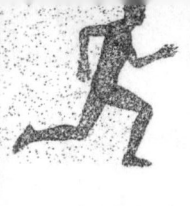

DAY TWO

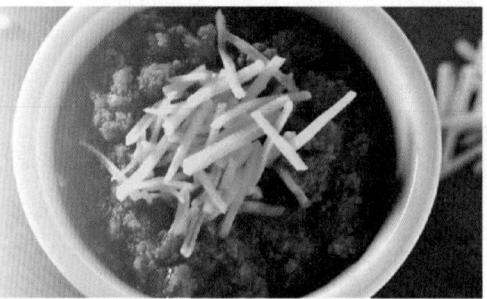

 Breakfast:
- 2 Eggs (any style)
- Bacon or sugar free sausage
- Coffee with heavy cream (& no-carb sweetener if desired)

Snack: Half an avocado with salt and pepper or cheese sticks

 Lunch:
- Simple tuna salad (tuna, mayonnaise or olive oil, salt and pepper)
- romaine lettuce leaves (just spoon it in and eat like a taco)
- fresh sliced jalapenos or bell peppers

Snack: Handful of almonds and/or 2 sticks of string cheese

 **Dinner:**
- Chili
- Cheddar cheese
- Sour cream

What is TSC Chili? Grass fed ground beef cooked/browned in a pan with taco seasoning plus cheese and sour cream.

Dessert:
½ cup full-fat Greek yogurt with 1 tablespoon almond butter and 1 tablespoon cocoa. Delicious!

 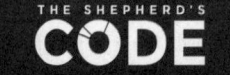

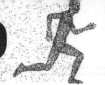

DAY THREE

 Breakfast:
- Cream Cheese Pancakes
- coffee with heavy cream and no-carb sweetener if desired
- Bacon or sugar-free breakfast sausage

 Snack: Handful of almonds and/or 2 sticks of string cheese

 Lunch:
Leftover chili, tuna salad, or ham and cheese/pancake rollups

 Snack:
- 1 cup chicken broth
- half an avocado with lite salt and pepper

 Dinner:
- Hamburger with bacon and cheddar cheese, wrapped in a large leaf of lettuce
- A small salad with your favorite high-fat dressing such as ranch, blue cheese or organic olive oil

In addition to these great quick-start meal plans you will also want to read our other four bonuses included in your purchase

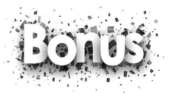

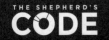

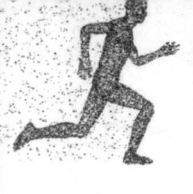
The Cellular Rejuvenation Secrets Manual—One of the main benefits of switching your body's fuel source from mainly sugars and carbohydrates to healthy fats is what is known as cellular rejuvenation. Cellular rejuvenation is what happens when "dying cells" in your body... are restored back to how they were when you were in your 20's. And once your cells are fully rejuvenated... you will look and feel younger.

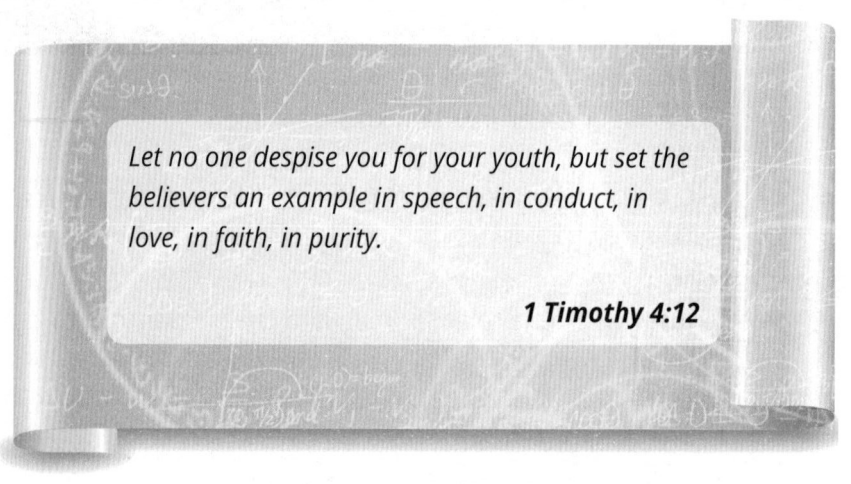

Let no one despise you for your youth, but set the believers an example in speech, in conduct, in love, in faith, in purity.

1 Timothy 4:12

Be ready for it... everyone will be asking you what you've done to suddenly look and feel so youthful! Be wary of the haters who are skeptical. Have patience with them and just show them the way!

The Anti-Anxiety & Stress Elimination Guide—Did you know that there are two emotions that virtually shut down the metabolic process and makes it almost impossible for you to lose weight? It's true! These emotions are anxiety and stress. The stress hormone in the body causes you to put on more weight, makes you insulin resistant and can even destroy your metabolic health... Which is why I'm going to share several simple techniques to help you reduce or eliminate anxiety and stress.

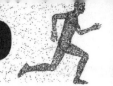

The Celebrity Anti-aging and Weight-loss Secret—You don't need to be a rich and famous celebrity to learn their secrets. After treating many esteemed **"private clients"** I have the answers to reveal to you... for free!

Once you start using the same "health boosting" secrets celebrities are using—which are far more focussed on "anti-aging" and looking younger... You'll experience:

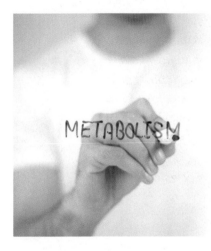

- A boost in metabolism... which helps you lose weight faster...

- A reduction in oxidative stress and inflammation which slows the signs of aging aging and reduces illness...

- Improved brain function...

  And much more...

Healthy Brain Manual—In this bonus, you'll get an incredible solution backed by the latest breakthroughs in scientific research that'll help you **HEAL YOUR BRAIN** and **enhance your focus and memory.**

You'll be smarter, sharper, and more mentally fit **in just 5 minutes a day**.

You'll discover exactly **how to give your MIND the nutrition it craves.**

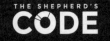

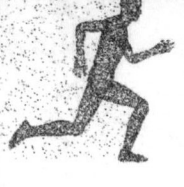
Finally, I want you to know that I am here for you. If you have questions or problems, please contact our customer service team at **support@theshepherdscode.com**

> *Two are better than one, because they have a good reward for their toil. For if they fall, one will lift up his fellow. But woe to him who is alone when he falls and has not another to lift him up! Again, if two lie together, they keep warm, but how can one keep warm alone? And though a man might prevail against one who is alone, two will withstand him—a threefold cord is not quickly broken.*
>
> ***Ecclesiastes 4:9-12***

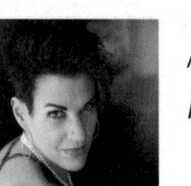

All things are possible!
Kristina Wilds

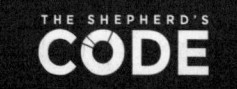

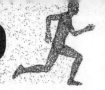

P.S. To access *The Shepherd's Code System* and purchased bonuses, including *Fat Loss Results Accelerator, Simple Body Sculpting System*, and/or *Wildfire Kitchen*... simply visit **www.shepcode.com/members**. Type in the email address you used to make your purchase and click the button to get instant access.

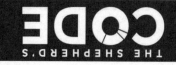

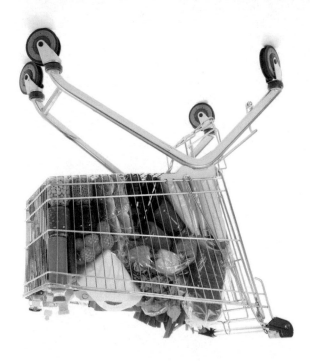

WHAT WOULD
JESUS EAT
GROCERY
FIELD GUIDE

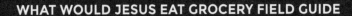
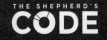

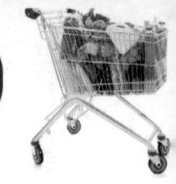

The contents of this document are based upon my opinions of *The Shepherd's Code* unless otherwise noted. This work is intended to share knowledge and information learned through research, experience, and discussions with others. The opinions of others, such as in the comments and the forum, are their own and are not endorsed by *The Shepherd's Code*. The information contained herein is not intended to diagnose, treat, cure or prevent any condition or disease, but rather to provide general information that is intended to be used for educational purposes only. Please consult with your physician or healthcare practitioner if you have any concerns. By using, viewing and interacting with *The Shepherd's Code* or **shepherdscode.com** website, you agree to all terms of engagement, thus assuming complete responsibility for your own actions. The authors and publishers will not claim accountability, nor shall they be held liable for any loss or injury sustained by you. Use, view and interact with these resources at your own risk. All products and information given to you by *The Shepherd's Code* and its related companies are strictly for informational purposes only. While every attempt has been made to verify the accuracy of information provided on our website and within our publications, neither the authors nor the publishers are responsible for assuming liability for possible inaccuracies. The authors and publishers disclaim any responsibility for the inaccuracy of the content, including but not limited to errors or omissions. Loss of property, injury to self or others, and even death could occur as a direct or indirect consequence of the use and application of any content found herein. Please act responsibly. The information provided may need to be downloaded and/or viewed using third party software, such as Acrobat. It's the user's responsibility to install the software necessary to view such information. Any downloads, whether purchased or given for free from our website, related websites or hosting systems are performed at the user's own risk. Although we take great preventative measures, we cannot warranty that our websites are free of corrupting computer codes, viruses or worms. If you are a minor, you can use this service only with permission and guidance from your parents or guardians.

And God said, "Behold, I have given you every plant yielding seed that is on the face of all the earth, and every tree with seed in its fruit. You shall have them for food.

Genesis 1:29

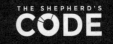

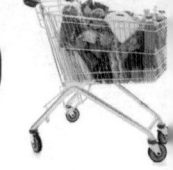

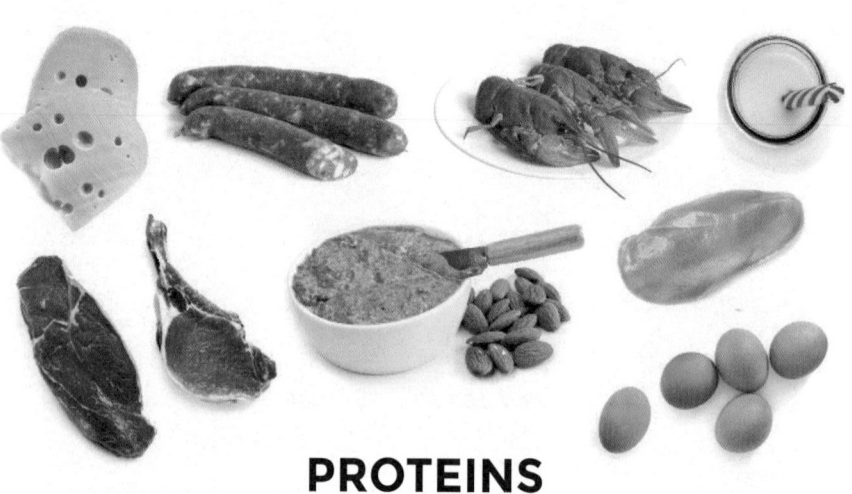

PROTEINS

- Anchovies
- Almond butter *(freshly ground)*
- Bacon *(not turkey bacon)*
- Beef jerky *(watch out for added sugars)*
- Beef ribs
- Beef roast
- Bratwurst
- Chicken organic *(choose the darkest cuts, skin on)*
- Cottage cheese 4%

- Duck
- Eggs *(whole)*
- Fish wild caught not farm raised —*(salmon, bass, carp, flounder, halibut, mackerel, sardines, trout)*
- Full-fat yogurt
- Ground beef *(grass fed)*
- Ham
- Kielbasa
- Lamb
- Pheasant
- Pork chops

- Pork ribs
- Pork rinds
- Pork roast
- Sausage
- Shellfish *(scallops, shrimp, crab meat, mussels, oysters)*
- Steak *(the fattier the better)*
- Tofu
- Tuna (in oil)
- Quail
- Turkey *(darker pieces are best)*
- Veal

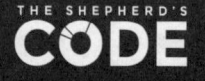

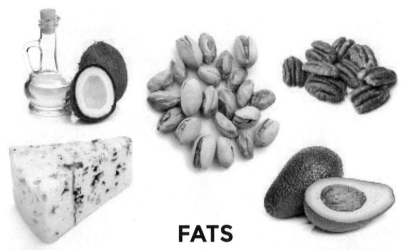

FATS

- Almonds
- Almond butter
- Almond milk, unsweetened
- Almond oil
- Avocado
- Avocado oil
- Bacon *(protein and fat)*
- Beef tallow
- Blue cheese
- Brazil nuts
- Butter grass fed
- Cheese full fat *(cheddar, Colby,*

feta, mozzarella, provolone, ricotta, Swiss, and others)
- Chicken fat
- Coconut
- Coconut cream
- Coconut milk, unsweetened
- Coconut oil
- Cream cheese
- Dark chocolate *(80 percent or higher)*
- Fish oil
- Ghee

- Full-fat Greek yogurt
- Heavy whipping cream
- Lard
- MCT oil
- Macadamia nut oil
- Macadamia nuts
- Olive oil organic
- Pecans
- Pili nuts
- Pistachios
- Sour cream
- Walnuts

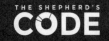

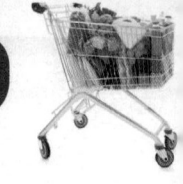

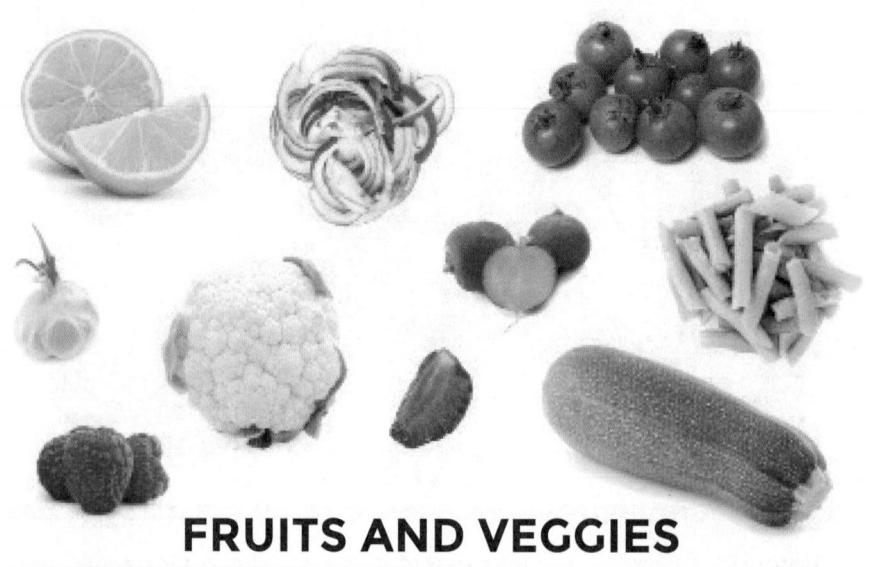

FRUITS AND VEGGIES

- Arugula
- Artichokes
- Asparagus
- Blackberries
- Blueberries
- Bok choy
- Broccoli
- Brussels sprouts
- Cabbage
- Cauliflower
- Celery
- Cucumbers
- Eggplant

- Garlic
- Green beans
- Kale
- Leeks
- Lemon
- Lettuce
- Lime
- Mushrooms
- Okra
- Onions
- Parsley
- Peppers
- Pumpkin

- Radicchio
- Radishes
- Raspberries
- Rhubarb
- Scallions
- Shallots
- Snow peas
- Spaghetti squash
- Spinach
- Strawberries
- Summer squash
- Tomatoes
- Zucchini

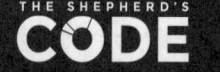

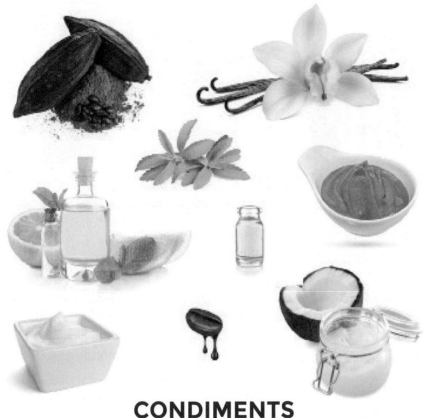

CONDIMENTS

- Cocoa
- Coconut extract
- Coffee extract
- Erythritol
- Lemon extract
- Mayonnaise
- Mustard

- Orange extract
- Stevia
- Strawberry extract
- Sugar-free chocolate syrup
- Swerve
- Truvia

- Vanilla extract
- Sugar-free maple syrup

 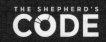

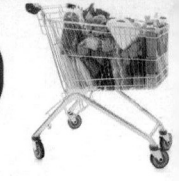

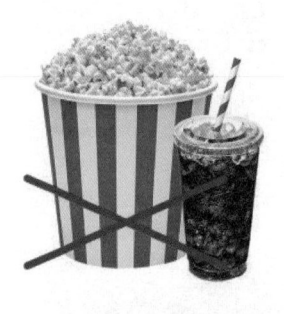
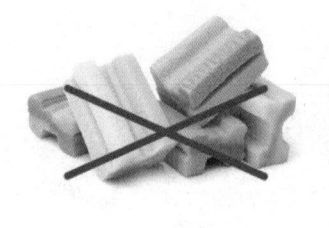
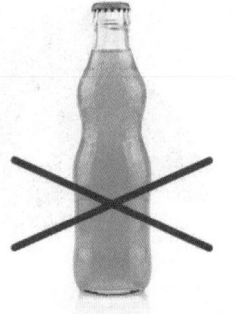

FOODS TO AVOID

- Refined sugar
- Sugar alcohols *(xylitol, malitol, and sorbitol that are found in chewing gums)*
- Alcohol
- Soda
- Grains

- Beans and legumes *(chickpeas, lentils, kidney beans)*
- Peanut butter with margarine/ substitute butter spreads
- Refined vegetable oils *(canola, peanut, sunflower;*

although vegetable oils are fats, they're heavily processed with chemicals and deodorizers, which makes them far from being healthy foods.)
- Low-fat diary products *(which are higher in carbs)*

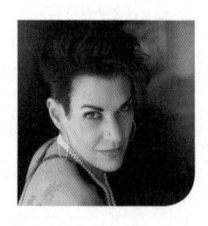

All things are possible!

Kristina Wilds

14-DAY EASY MEAL PLANS

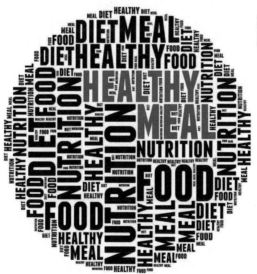

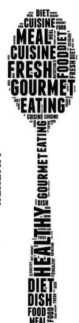

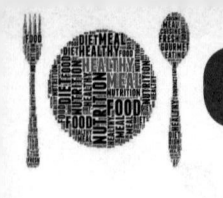

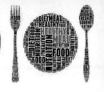

The contents of this document are based upon my opinions of *The Shepherd's Code* unless otherwise noted. This work is intended to share knowledge and information learned through research, experience, and discussions with others. The opinions of others, such as in the comments and the forum, are their own and are not endorsed by *The Shepherd's Code*. The information contained herein is not intended to diagnose, treat, cure or prevent any condition or disease, but rather to provide general information that is intended to be used for educational purposes only. Please consult with your physician or healthcare practitioner if you have any concerns. By using, viewing and interacting with *The Shepherd's Code* or **shepherdscode.com** website, you agree to all terms of engagement, thus assuming complete responsibility for your own actions. The authors and publishers will not claim accountability, nor shall they be held liable for any loss or injury sustained by you. Use, view and interact with these resources at your own risk. All products and information given to you by *The Shepherd's Code* and its related companies are strictly for informational purposes only. While every attempt has been made to verify the accuracy of information provided on our website and within our publications, neither the authors nor the publishers are responsible for assuming liability for possible inaccuracies. The authors and publishers disclaim any responsibility for the inaccuracy of the content, including but not limited to errors or omissions. Loss of property, injury to self or others, and even death could occur as a direct or indirect consequence of the use and application of any content found herein. Please act responsibly. The information provided may need to be downloaded and/or viewed using third party software, such as Acrobat. It's the user's responsibility to install the software necessary to view such information. Any downloads, whether purchased or given for free from our website, related websites or hosting systems are performed at the user's own risk. Although we take great preventative measures, we cannot warranty that our websites are free of corrupting computer codes, viruses or worms. If you are a minor, you can use this service only with permission and guidance from your parents or guardians.

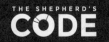

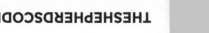

4

BREAKFAST

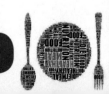

14-DAY EASY MEAL PLANS

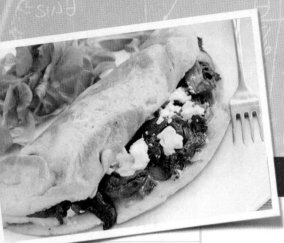

FETA SPINACH OMELET

SERVES: 1 - PREP: 15 MINS.

INGREDIENTS

- [ ] Large eggs 3
- [ ] Feta cheese 2 oz
- [ ] Garlic clove 1
- [ ] Mushrooms 3 oz
- [ ] Fresh spinach 3 oz
- [ ] Purified butter 2 tbsp
- [ ] Fresh coriander 2 tbsp
- [ ] Salt and pepper to taste

PREPARATION

1. For filling: First, finely dice the garlic and place in a pan *(greased with a tablespoon of ghee). Sprinkle with salt and* cook over a medium-high heat for just a minute *until fragrant.*

2. Add sliced mushrooms and cook until lightly browned *(approximately 5 minutes, stirring occasionally).*

3. Add spinach and cook for one minute. When done, transfer to a bowl *and discard excess liquid.*

4. Crack the eggs into a bowl and mix by fork. *Season with salt and pepper to taste.*

5. Pour the eggs evenly in a hot pan. *(greased with ghee).*

6. When the top is almost cooked, add the spinach and mushroom topping and crumbled feta. Fold the omelet in half.

7. Cook for another minute just to warm up the topping *(slide on a serving plate).*

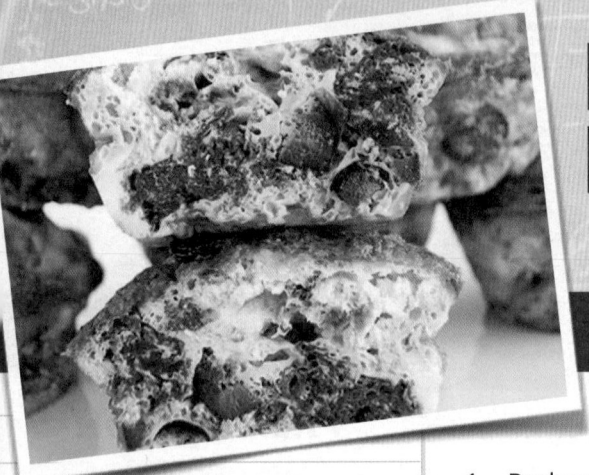

EGG PESTO MUFFINS

PREPARATION

1. Preheat the oven to 350F.

2. Squeeze out the excess water from the spinach, slice the olives, and chop the sun-dried tomatoes.

3. In separate bowl, crack the eggs, add the pesto and season with salt and pepper to taste. Mix until well combined.

4. Divide the spinach, crumbled goat cheese, sun-dried tomatoes, and olives evenly into a muffin pan.

5. Pour in the egg and pesto mixture and transfer into the oven.

6. Bake for 20-25 minutes or until browned on top.

7. Remove from the oven and set aside to cool down.

8. These can be stored in the fridge for up to 5 days.

INGREDIENTS

- ☐ Frozen spinach 4 oz
- ☐ Pesto 2 oz
- ☐ Olives ¼ cup
- ☐ Chopped sun-dried toma-toes 2 tbsp
- ☐ Goat cheese 8 oz
- ☐ Large eggs 6
- ☐ Salt and pepper to taste

THE SHEPHERD'S
C♦DE

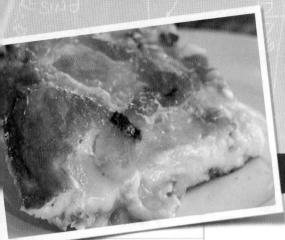

BACON BRIE FRITTATA

SERVES: 6 - PREP: 20 MINS.

INGREDIENTS

- [ ] Bacon 8 slices chopped
- [ ] Large eggs 8
- [ ] Whipping cream 3/8 cup
- [ ] Garlic cloves 2
- [ ] Salt and pepper to taste
- [ ] Brie cheese 4 oz

PREPARATION

1. Cook chopped bacon in a pan over medium heat until crispy. Set aside.

2. In a large bowl, mix eggs with cream, garlic, salt and pepper, and about two thirds of the cooked bacon.

3. Transfer egg mixture to the pan and cook undisturbed for about 10 minutes.

4. Lay slices of brie on top of frittata and sprinkle with remaining bacon.

5. Continue to cook until puffed and golden brown, about 5 minutes.

6. Remove and let cool for a minute or two before serving.

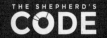

COCONUT FAT BOMBS

SERVES: 10 - PREP: 15 MINS.

INGREDIENTS

- [ ] Coconut oil 3.5 fl oz
- [ ] Heavy whipped cream ½ cup
- [ ] Cream cheese ½ cup
- [ ] Pineapple extract 1 tsp
- [ ] Stevia 10 drops
- [ ] Protein powder 2 tbsp

PREPARATION

1. Mix coconut oil, heavy cream, and cream cheese. Using mixer, mix all the ingredients together or place in microwave oven for 30 seconds to 1 minute to soften them.

2. Add pineapple extract and liquid stevia to the mixture and mix with a spoon.

3. Distribute the mixture into a silicone ice-cube tray and freeze for 3 hours.

4. Goes great with coffee!

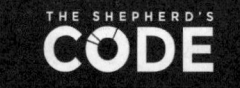

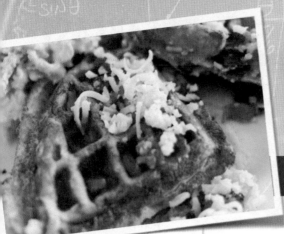

CHEDDAR WAFFLES

SERVES: 12 - PREP: 15 MINS.

PREPARATION

1. Preheat your waffle maker.

2. In a mixing bowl, whisk flour, baking powder, and seasonings together.

3. Add your liquid ingredients and mix until stiff batter forms.

4. Mix in the cheese.

5. When your machine is warm, grease it, then pour batter into the machine and cook until steam rises, or until the top panel opens freely without sticking to the waffle.

INGREDIENTS

- ☐ Coconut flour 1 ¼ cup
- ☐ Coconut milk 2 cups
- ☐ Melted coconut-oil 3 tbsp
- ☐ Cheddar cheese 8 oz
- ☐ Eggs 2
- ☐ Baking powder 3 tsp.
- ☐ Dried sage powder 1 tsp
- ☐ Salt to taste
- ☐ Garlic powder to taste
- ☐ Water ½ cup

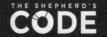

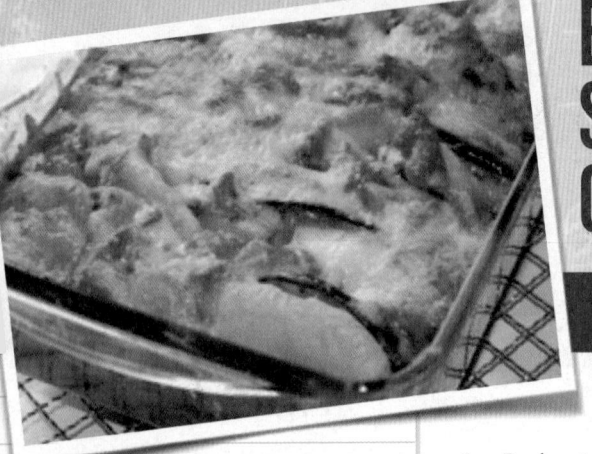

BREAKFAST SAUSAGE CASSEROLE

SERVES: 6 - PREP: 45 MINS.

INGREDIENTS

- [ ] Pork sausage 1 lb
- [ ] Diced zucchini 1 lb
- [ ] Green cabbage 1 lb
- [ ] Diced onion 4 oz
- [ ] Eggs 3
- [ ] Mayonnaise ½ cup
- [ ] Yellow mustard 2 tsp
- [ ] Dried ground sage 1 tsp
- [ ] Cheddar cheese 10 oz
- [ ] Parmesan 1 oz
- [ ] Cayenne pepper to taste

PREPARATION

1. Preheat oven to 375F.

2. Grease a casserole dish and set aside.

3. In a large skillet, brown sausage over medium heat until almost cooked through.

4. Add cabbage, zucchini, onion and cook until vegetables are tender.

5. Move contents from the skillet to the casserole dish.

6. In a separate bowl, whisk eggs, mayonnaise, mustard, sage, and pepper until smooth. Add grated cheeses (cheddar and Parmesan) to the egg mixture and stir.

7. Pour this mixture over the top of sausage and vegetables in the casserole dish.

8. Place casserole dish in preheated oven and bake for 30 minutes or until cheese is melted and lightly browned on top. Serve immediately.

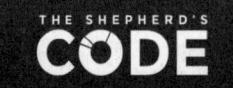
THE SHEPHERD'S
CODE

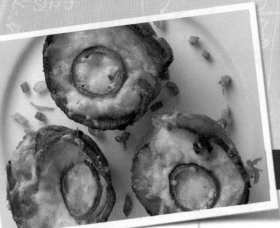

PEPPER EGG CUPS

SERVES: 3 - PREP: 15 MINS.

INGREDIENTS

- ☐ Bacon 12 strips
- ☐ Eggs 8
- ☐ Cheddar cheese ½ cup
- ☐ Cream cheese 3/8 cup
- ☐ Jalapeño peppers 4
- ☐ Garlic powder ½ tsp
- ☐ Onion powder ½ tsp
- ☐ Salt and pepper (as needed)

PREPARATION

1. Preheat oven to 375F.

2. Slice 1 jalapeño into rings as a garnish for the top. Cook bacon so it's semi crisp but still pliable. Save bacon grease in the pan.

3. Using a hand mixer, mix together eggs, cream cheese, 3 chopped and seeded jalapeño peppers, leftover bacon grease, garlic powder, onion powder, and salt and pepper to taste.

4. Grease muffin tin, then place cooked bacon around the edges forming a cup.

5. Pour egg mixture into the muffin tin. Make sure you only go about 2/3 way up as they rise quite a lot.

6. Add grated cheddar cheese on the top of the muffin, then add jalapeño rings.

7. Cook at 375F for 20-25 minutes. Once cooked, remove from the oven to let cool.

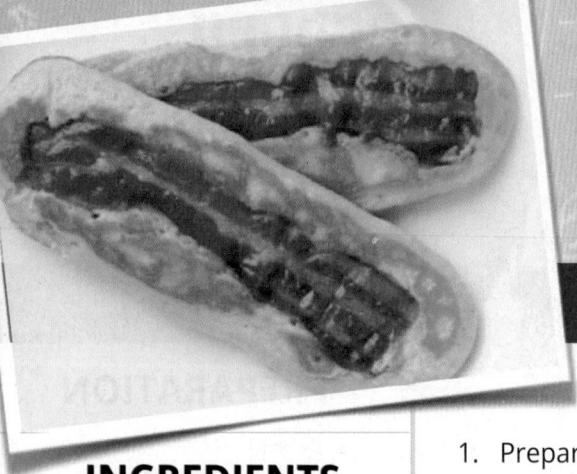

BACON STUFFED PANCAKES

SERVES: 2 - PREP: 30 MINS.

PREPARATION

1. Prepare the crispy bacon by placing in oven (375F) for 15 minutes, until the bacon is crisp.

2. For making pancakes, combine all pancake ingredients into a bowl and mix well.

3. Heat a large pan and grease with ghee. When ghee is hot, pour the batter and top with a slice of crispy bacon. Cook for 5 minutes each side, or until golden.

4. Meanwhile, make chocolate dip by mixing all ingredients. Serve with each pancake.

INGREDIENTS

Pancake:

- ☐ Thin bacon slices 8
- ☐ Coconut flour 2 oz
- ☐ Almond flour 6 oz
- ☐ Protein 1 tbsp
- ☐ Swerve 2 oz
- ☐ Baking soda 1/2 tsp
- ☐ Cream of tartar 1 tsp
- ☐ Eggs 4
- ☐ Ghee 2 fl oz
- ☐ Almond milk 16 fl oz
- ☐ Liquid stevia 10 drops

Chocolate dip:

- ☐ Cocoa powder 2 tbsp
- ☐ Ghee 2 tbsp
- ☐ Swerve 2 tbsp

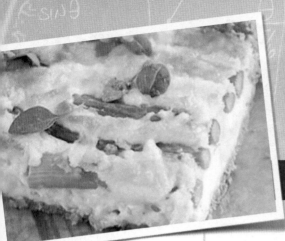

PORK AND ASPARAGUS QUICHE

SERVES: 8 - PREP: 60 MINS.

PREPARATION

1. Preheat the oven to 400F.
2. Powder the pork rinds *in a food processor or blender.*
3. Add all crust ingredients to a bowl and mix until a dough is formed.
4. Place dough in a rectangular baking tray *with removable bottom.*
5. Bake for 15 minutes, then set aside to cool. Reduce the oven to 350F.
6. While baking, take a large bowl and crack the eggs, add the cream, *season with salt and pepper, and whisk until well combined.*
7. Place a pan over medium heat with ghee. When ghee is hot, add sliced spring onions and cook for 3 minutes or until fragrant.
8. Add onions to the egg mixture *and combine well.*
9. Add cream cheese to egg mixture. *Sprinkle shredded cheddar and mascarpone cheeses on the crust,* then pour the egg mixture over the shredded cheese.
10. Now, top egg mixture with asparagus and place in oven for 30 minutes *or until lightly browned and crispy on top.*
11. Garnish with freshly chopped herbs and serve.

INGREDIENTS

Crust:

- [ ] Pork rinds 5 oz
- [ ] Coconut flour 5 oz
- [ ] Flax meal 3 tbsp
- [ ] Large eggs 3
- [ ] Himalayan sea salt 1/2 tsp

Filling:

- [ ] Large eggs 6
- [ ] Heavy whipping cream 4 fl oz
- [ ] Spring onions 1 oz
- [ ] Cheddar cheese 7 oz
- [ ] Mascarpone cheese 4 oz
- [ ] Cream cheese 9 oz
- [ ] Asparagus spears 9 oz
- [ ] Salt and pepper to taste
- [ ] Fresh herbs for garnish
- [ ] Ghee 1 tbsp

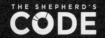

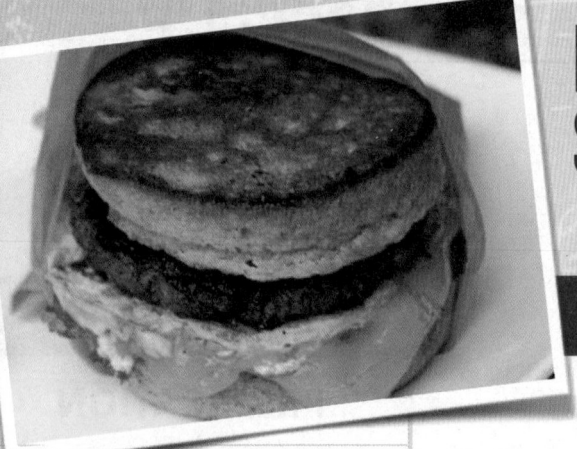

BREAKFAST SANDWICH

SERVES: 1 - PREP: 15 MINS.

INGREDIENTS

Bun:

- ☐ Ground pork rinds 5 tsp
- ☐ Almond flour 1 tbsp
- ☐ Egg 1
- ☐ Heavy cream 1 tbsp
- ☐ Vanilla extract ½ tsp
- ☐ Maple syrup 2 tbsp

Filling:

- ☐ Hot sausage 2 oz
- ☐ Cheddar cheese 1 slice
- ☐ Egg 1

PREPARATION

1. Heat a pan to medium high heat.

2. Form sausage into patties and cook until done.

3. While sausage is cooking, mix together ground pork rinds with all pancake bun ingredients.

4. Put an egg ring mold inside the pan and fill 3/4 of the way with bun batter, so that the bun cooks like a biscuit.

5. Once the bun is browned on the bottom, remove the ring mold and flip to the other side. Cook until both sides are browned.

6. In the same pan, add an egg to the ring mold and lightly scramble. Cook completely until solidified.

7. Assemble together with 1 bun on bottom, 1 slice of cheese, egg, sausage, and the last bun on top. Then serve.

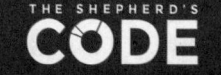

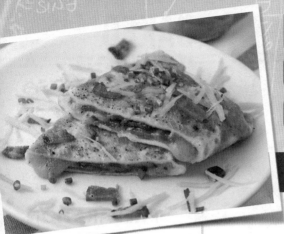

BACON CHEDDAR OMELETTE

SERVES: 1 - TIME: 15 MINS.

INGREDIENTS

- ☐ Cooked bacon 2 slices
- ☐ Eggs 2
- ☐ Cheddar cheese 9 oz
- ☐ Chives 2 stems
- ☐ Salt and pepper (as needed)

PREPARATION

1. Fry the bacon in a pan. While it's cooking, shred the cheese and chop the chives.

2. When the bacon reaches your desired crispiness, set it aside on a paper towel. Leave the bacon grease in the pan.

3. Season the eggs with salt and pepper as desired, then whisk vigorously.

4. Pour them into the pan with the bacon grease, swirling so that it fills the whole pan.

5. When the edges begin to pull away from the sides, carefully flip the omelette.

6. After flipping, add the chives, cheese, and chopped bacon pieces to one side of the omelette. When the cheese is melted, carefully fold the omelette in half.

7. Enjoy!

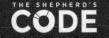

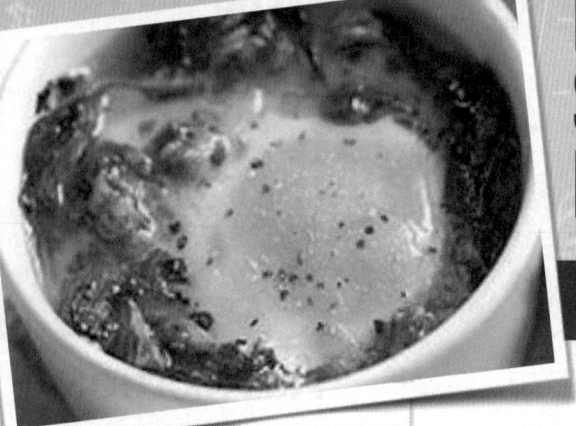

BAKED SPINACH EGGS

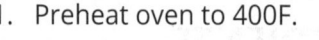

SERVES: 4 - PREP: 25 MINS.

INGREDIENTS

- [ ] Olive oil 2 tsp
- [ ] Diced shallots 2 tbsp
- [ ] Spinach 1.5 lb
- [ ] Large eggs 4
- [ ] Purified butter 1 ½ tbsp
- [ ] Salt to taste
- [ ] Fresh ground pepper to taste
- [ ] Grated Asiago cheese 2 tbsp
- [ ] Mascarpone cheese 2 tbsp
- [ ] Grated coconut 2 tbsp

PREPARATION

1. Preheat oven to 400F.

2. Grease ramekins with butter.

3. Heat a large pan over medium-low heat, add olive oil and shallots and cook 2 minutes.

4. Add spinach, salt, and pepper and saute until the spinach wilts— about 3 minutes. Mix in cheeses and remove from heat.

5. Divide the spinach into ramekins and make a hollow opening in the center.

6. Crack an egg into the hole and season with grated coconut, salt, and pepper.

7. Place the ramekins on a baking sheet and bake until the white is set and the yolks are tight around the edges but still soft in the middle- about 17 minutes.

8. Serve immediately.

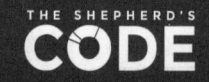

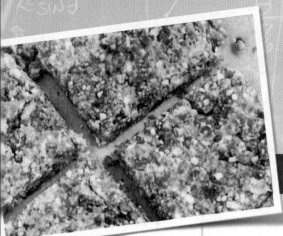

COCONUT CASHEW BAR

SERVES: 8 - PREP: 15 MINS.

PREPARATION

1. Combine almond flour and melted butter in a large bowl. Add cinnamon, salt, maple syrup, and protein powder and mix well.

2. Add crushed coconut and mix again. Add chopped almond nuts and mix everything evenly.

3. Line a casserole with parchment paper and spread the dough in a flat layer. Sprinkle crushed coconut and cinnamon on top for a crispy texture and flavor.

4. Place in refrigerator and cool overnight. Cut into bars and serve.

INGREDIENTS

- [ ] Almond flour 1 cup
- [ ] Butter 2 fl oz
- [ ] Maple syrup 1 oz
- [ ] Cinnamon 1 tsp
- [ ] Salt to taste
- [ ] Almond nuts 3/8 cup
- [ ] Protein powder 2 oz
- [ ] Shredded coconut 1 tbsp

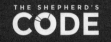

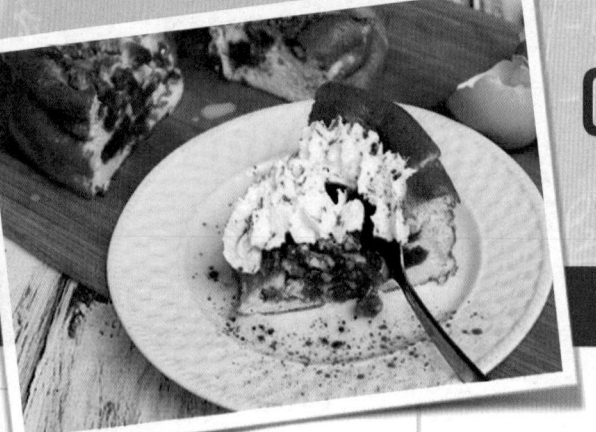

COFFEE CAKE

INGREDIENTS

Base:

- [ ] Eggs 6
- [ ] Cream cheese 6 oz
- [ ] Erythritol 1.5 oz
- [ ] Liquid stevia 1 tsp
- [ ] Protein powder 2 tbsp
- [ ] Vanilla extract 2 tsp
- [ ] Cream of tartar 1 tsp

Filling:

- [ ] Almond flour 1 cup
- [ ] Cinnamon 1 tsp
- [ ] Butter ½ cup
- [ ] Maple syrup 2.5 tbsp
- [ ] Erythritol 1 oz

PREPARATION

1. Preheat your oven to 325F.

2. In a bowl, add egg yolks, erythritol, and liquid stevia. Mix well until it looks creamy, then add cream cheese and protein powder. Mix this together well until a thick batter forms.

3. Beat your egg whites together with the cream of tartar until stiff peaks form.

4. Fold the egg whites into the egg yolk mixture and pour the batter into a round cake pan.

5. Mix together all of the filling ingredients and put in the cake pan. Bake for 20 minutes and then top with the rest of the cinnamon filling.

6. Bake for another 20-30 minutes until a toothpick comes out clean. Let cool for 20 minutes before removing from the cake pan.

7. Top with whipped cream if desired and serve.

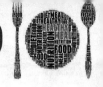

LUNCH

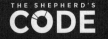

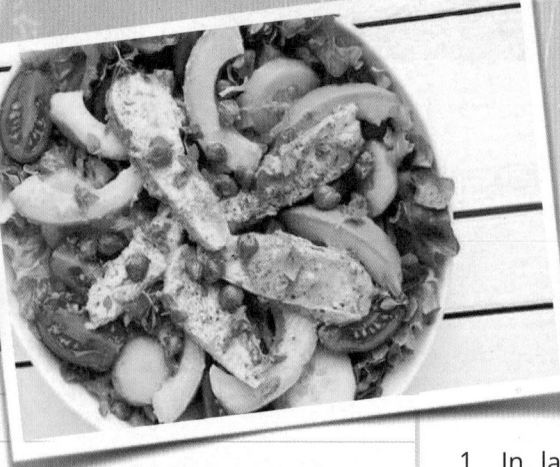

PESTO CHICKEN SALAD

SERVES: 8 - PREP: 15 MINS.

PREPARATION

1. In large bowl, combine chicken, bacon, chayote squash, tomatoes, mayonnaise and pesto. Mix gently to coat.

2. Rip up lettuce leaves and serve the chicken on top as a salad, or keep the leaves intact and roll up the chicken and serve as lettuce wraps.

INGREDIENTS

- ☐ Chicken, cooked and cubed 2 lbs
- ☐ Bacon, cooked crisp and crumbled 12 slices
- ☐ Medium chayote squash, cubed 2
- ☐ Grape tomatoes, halved 20
- ☐ Mayonnaise 1/2 cup
- ☐ Garlic pesto 4 tablespoons
- ☐ Several fresh butter lettuce leaves

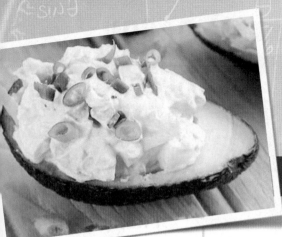

EGG STUFFED AVOCADO

SERVES: 2 - PREP: 15 MINS.

PREPARATION

1. Begin by hard boiling the eggs. This can be done ahead of time.

2. Dice the eggs and slice the spring onion.

3. In a bowl, mix the diced eggs, mayo, sour cream, mustard, and spring onion. Keep some spring onion for garnish. Season with salt and pepper to taste.

4. Cut the avocados in half and scoop out the flesh. Cut into small pieces and combine with the egg mixture.

5. Finally, fill each avocado half with the egg and avocado mixture and top with sliced spring onion.

INGREDIENTS

- [ ] Avocados 2 (seed removed)
- [ ] Large eggs 4 large
- [ ] Mayonnaise ¼ cup
- [ ] Sour cream 2 tbsp
- [ ] Dijon mustard 1 tsp
- [ ] Spring onions 2 tbsp
- [ ] Sea salt to taste
- [ ] Freshly ground black pepper

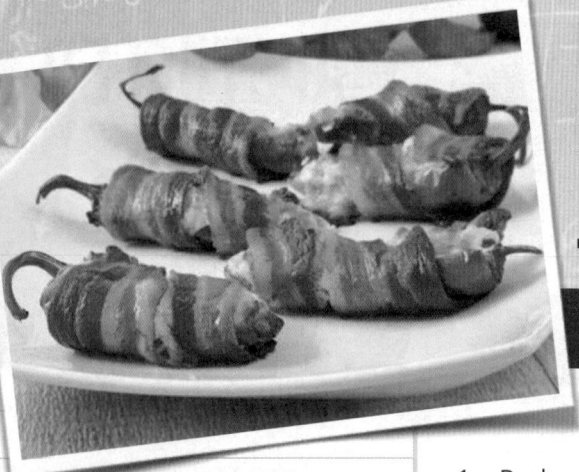

BACON ROLLED JALAPEÑO

SERVES: 4 - PREP: 35 MINS.

PREPARATION

1. Preheat the oven to 400F.

2. Wash the jalapeños and clean with paper towel. Halve and de-seed the jalapeños.

3. Mix the grated Gruyere cheese, ricotta, and finely chopped cilantro and fill each jalapeño half with the cheese mixture.

4. Wrap each jalapeño half with a bacon slice and place on a baking sheet lined with parchment paper.

5. Bake for 20-25 minutes until golden and crispy.

6. Can be served hot or cold.

INGREDIENTS

- [ ] Jalapeño peppers 12 (0.4 lb)
- [ ] Ricotta cheese 1 cup
- [ ] Gruyere cheese ¼ cup
- [ ] Bacon slices 12 (0.8 lb)
- [ ] Freshly chopped cilantro 2 tbsp

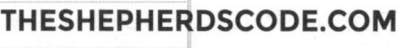

THE SHEPHERD'S
CODE

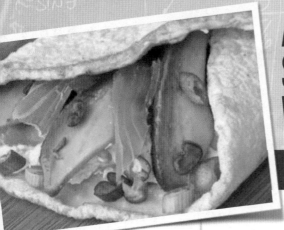

AVOCADO SALMON WRAPS

INGREDIENTS

- ☐ Large eggs 3
- ☐ Avocado 3 oz
- ☐ Smoked salmon 2 oz
- ☐ Cream cheese 2 tbsp
- ☐ Fresh chives or spring onions 2 tbsp
- ☐ Salt and pepper to taste

PREPARATION

1. Choose your favorite low-carb tortilla, such as La Tortilla from netrition.com. Or for a simple alternative, make a thin egg "pancake" by whisking an egg and pouring into a hot pan. When the edges of the egg start to pull up, it's ready to flip. This way you can keep it together as one sheet.

2. Slice the smoked salmon and avocado.

3. Spread the cream cheese on your tortilla, sprinkle chives or green onions on top, and top with salmon and avocado.

4. Roll up and serve!

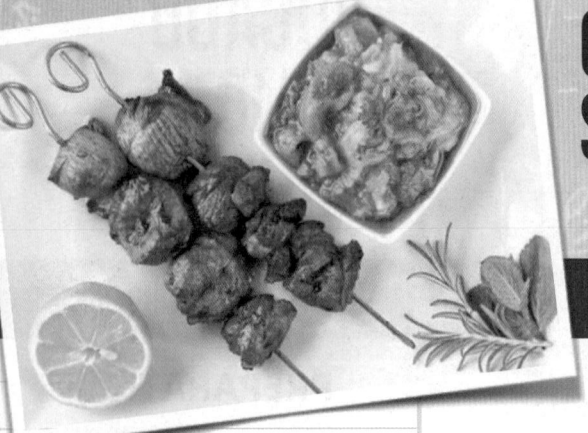

GREEK LAMB SKEWERS

SERVES: 4 - PREP: 50 MINS.

PREPARATION

1. Preheat the oven to 450F.

2. Place in a bowl and add extra virgin olive oil and freshly juiced lemon. Finely chop the mint and rosemary and add to the bowl.

3. Season with salt and mix well to cover the meat in the oil mixture on all sides. Keep in the fridge for 4 hours or overnight.

4. Slice the meat into medium sized pieces.

5. Put the skewers through each meat cube and place them in oven to cook for 15 minutes. Turning the skewers and cook for another 10 minutes

6. When it looks crispy and browned, remove from the oven and let them cool.

7. Serve immediately with fresh vegetable salad.

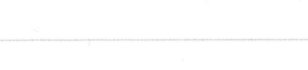

INGREDIENTS

- ☐ Boneless lamb 1.7 lb
- ☐ Chopped mint 3 tbsp
- ☐ Chopped rosemary 2 tbsp
- ☐ Lemon juice 3 tbsp
- ☐ Extra virgin olive oil 2 fl oz
- ☐ Salt to taste

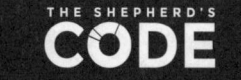

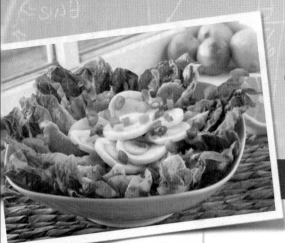

ROMAINE TUNA SALAD

SERVES: 1 - PREP: 5 MINS.

INGREDIENTS

- ☐ Head lettuce 4 oz
- ☐ Tuna 1 can
- ☐ Hard-boiled eggs 2
- ☐ Mayonnaise 1 oz
- ☐ Bunch chives 1 tbsp
- ☐ Lemon juice 1 tbsp
- ☐ Extra virgin olive oil 1 tbsp
- ☐ Salt to taste

PREPARATION

1. Tear the leaves of the romaine lettuce, then wash and drain in a salad spinner or with a paper towel. Spread the leaves over the bottom of a serving bowl.

2. Add drained and shredded tuna, then top with hard-boiled eggs, mayonnaise, and freshly chopped chives.

3. Drizzle with extra virgin olive oil and serve.

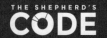

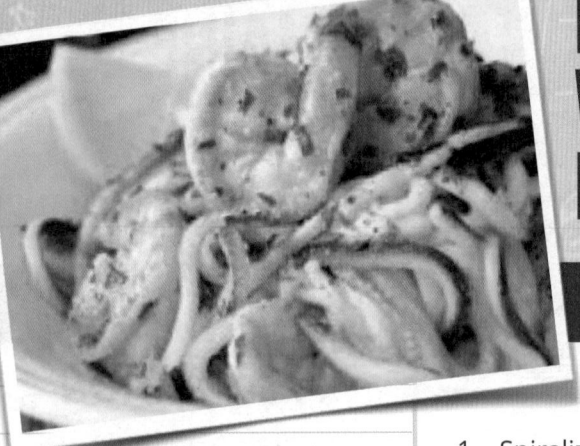

LEMON SHRIMP WITH ZUCCHINI NOODLES

SERVES: 4 - PREP: 30 MINS.

PREPARATION

1. Spiralize the zucchinis, cook in ghee on medium heat for ~5 minutes or until they reach your desired tenderness, then set aside.

2. Next, sauté the garlic in ghee for about 2 minutes, then add the shrimp and cook until they turn pink, about 3-5 minutes.

3. Add the noodles back into the pan. Pour the lemon juice on top and toss, then cook for 1 minute longer.

4. Serve and enjoy!

INGREDIENTS

- [ ] Zoodles 3 zucchinis
- [ ] Shrimp 1 lb.
- [ ] Minced garlic 2 tbsp.
- [ ] Ghee 2 tbsp
- [ ] Lemon juice 2 tbsp

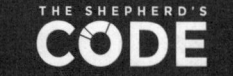

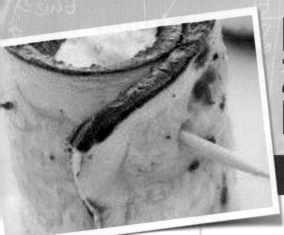

BACON ZUCCHINI ROLLS

INGREDIENTS

- [ ] Baby zucchini 8 oz
- [ ] Bacon 6 pieces
- [ ] Goat cheese 7 oz
- [ ] Sun-dried tomatoes 2 oz
- [ ] Apple cider vinegar 4 tbsp
- [ ] Fresh basil 2 tbsp

PREPARATION

1. Preheat your oven to 400F.

2. Using a peeler, slice the zucchini into thin strips. Put in a bowl and add the vinegar. Make sure you cover the zucchini on both sides. Let marinate for 10 minutes.

3. Cook bacon, but not too crispy. Make sure it's still pliable so you can roll it in the zucchini.

4. Place a bacon strip onto each zucchini slice. Top with soft goat cheese, a small piece of sun-dried tomato, and freshly chopped basil.

5. Wrap the zucchini rolls and pin each closed with a toothpick.

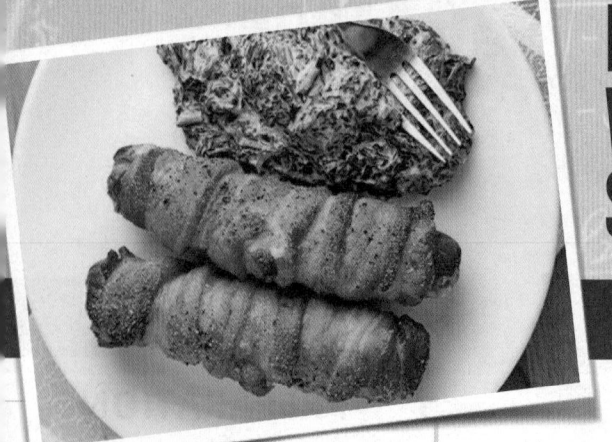

BACON WRAPPED SAUSAGES

SERVES: 6 - PREP: 45 MINS.

INGREDIENTS

- [ ] Sausages or hot dogs 6 (choose franks that are all natural and free of nitrates, or organic sausages)
- [ ] Bacon 12 slices
- [ ] Cheddar cheese ¼ cup
- [ ] Garlic powder ½ tsp
- [ ] Onion powder ½ tsp
- [ ] Salt and pepper (as needed)

PREPARATION

1. Pre-heat oven to 400F.

2. Make a slit in all of the hot dogs to make room for the cheese.

3. Slice cheddar cheese from a block into small long rectangles and stuff into the hot dogs.

4. Start by tightly wrapping one slice of bacon around the hot dog. Continue tightly wrapping the second slice of bacon around the hot dog, slightly overlapping with the first slice.

5. Poke toothpicks through each side of the bacon and hot dog, securing the bacon in place.

6. Set on a wire rack that's on top of a cookie sheet. Season with garlic powder, onion powder, salt and pepper.

7. Bake for 35-40 minutes, or until bacon is crispy. Additionally broil the bacon on top if needed. Serve up with some delicious creamed spinach.

THE SHEPHERD'S
CODE

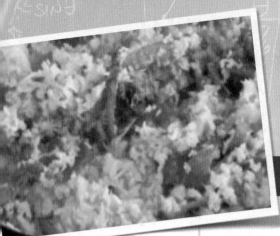

MEXICAN CHORIZO RICE

SERVES: 4 - PREP: 20 MINS.

INGREDIENTS

- ☐ Cauliflower rice 1 head
- ☐ Chorizo (or pepperoni if not available) 8 oz
- ☐ Jalapeńo peppers 3 oz
- ☐ Dry red chili 1
- ☐ Fresh cilantro 4 tbsp
- ☐ Ghee 2 tbsp
- ☐ Salt and pepper to taste

PREPARATION

1. Rice the cauliflower by using a food processor or blender. Set aside.

2. Slice chorizo, jalapeńo peppers, dry red chili, and keep aside.

3. Now, place a large skillet over medium heat and add ghee. When ghee is hot, add peppers, chili, and pepperoni. Cook until slightly browned.

4. Add the cauliflower rice and cook for 10 minutes, then season with salt and pepper.

5. When done, add finely chopped parsley and serve.

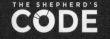

THAI BBQ-PORK SALAD

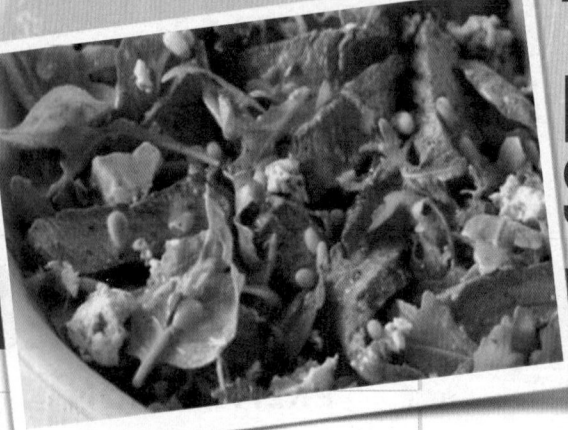

SERVES: 4 - PREP: 10 MINS.

INGREDIENTS

- ☐ Coconut oil 2 tablespoons
- ☐ Ground pork 2 lbs
- ☐ Large handful mixed minced herbs such as Thai basil, mint, cilantro
- ☐ Fresh ginger, minced 4- inch piece
- ☐ Garlic, minced 6 cloves
- ☐ Small shallots, thinly sliced 4
- ☐ Green onions, thinly sliced 8
- ☐ Fish sauce 2 tablespoons
- ☐ Coconut aminos 2 tsp
- ☐ zest of 1 lime
- ☐ juice of 1 lime
- ☐ red pepper flakes 2 tsp
- ☐ white pepper 1 tsp
- ☐ lettuce cups, for serving

PREPARATION

1. Heat the coconut oil in a large skillet over high heat.

2. Add the pork and shallots, cook 6-8 minutes, breaking the pork into small pieces.

3. While the pork is cooking, mix chopped garlic, chopped ginger, herbs, and green onions in a bowl.

4. In a second bowl mix fish sauce, coconut aminos, lemon juice and zest, red pepper flakes, and white pepper.

5. Add the herb mixture to the saucepan and cook for 1 minute. Next add the sauce and mix and cook for 1 minute.

6. Serve over the top of the lettuce as a salad, or wrapped up as lettuce wraps.

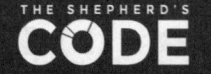

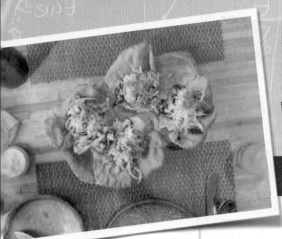

BUTTER LETTUCE WRAPS

INGREDIENTS

- [ ] Ground beef 1 lb
- [ ] Butter lettuce 1 head
- [ ] Soy sauce 2 tbsp
- [ ] Onions 1/2 cup
- [ ] Coconut oil 2 tbsp
- [ ] Sour cream 4 tbsp
- [ ] Cheese 4 oz
- [ ] Hot sauce

PREPARATION

1. Chop the onion and sauté in coconut oil until it's translucent. Then add the ground beef, pour in the soy sauce, and cook until brown.

2. Tear off lettuce leaves and stack them on a plate.

3. To serve, spoon the ground beef into each lettuce cup and eat it like a taco. Top with sour cream, cheese, and hot sauce.

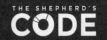

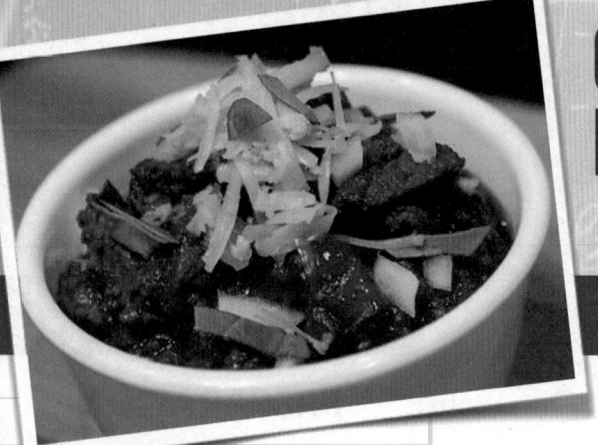

CHILI MEAT CUP

INGREDIENTS

- ☐ Ground beef 2 lb
- ☐ Onion 3 oz
- ☐ Green pepper 3 oz
- ☐ Beef broth 1 cup
- ☐ Tomato paste 1.5 oz
- ☐ Soy sauce 2 tbsp
- ☐ Olive oil 2 tbsp
- ☐ Chili powder 1 oz
- ☐ Cumin 1.5 tsp
- ☐ Fish sauce 1 tsp
- ☐ Minced garlic 1.5 tsp
- ☐ Paprika 1.5 tsp
- ☐ Oregano 1 tsp
- ☐ Cayenne pepper 1 tsp
- ☐ Worcestershire 1 tsp
- ☐ Black pepper 1 tsp
- ☐ Salt (as needed)

PREPARATION

1. Chop the onions and pepper into small pieces.

2. To a bowl, add beef broth, tomato paste, soy sauce, chili powder, cumin, fish sauce, minced garlic, paprika, oregano, cayenne pepper, Worcestershire and mix well.

3. In a pan, heat olive oil and begin cooking ground beef.

4. When beef is browned, add the broth/paste mixture.

5. After 10 minutes, add chopped pepper, onion, pepper, salt and seasonings.

6. Cook for 25 minutes and serve hot with cheese.

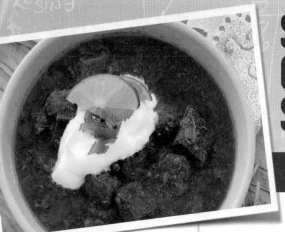

SLOW COOKER STEAK CHILI

SERVES: 12 - TIME: 6 HRS.

INGREDIENTS

Chili:

- [ ] Grass fed steak 2.5 lb
- [ ] Chili powder 1 tbsp
- [ ] Ground cumin 1 tsp
- [ ] Salt (as needed)
- [ ] Ground cayenne pepper ¼ tsp
- [ ] Ground black pepper ¼ tsp
- [ ] Leeks 3 oz
- [ ] Canned tomatoes 1 can
- [ ] Chicken or beef stock 8 oz

Topping:

- [ ] Cheddar cheese 2 tbsp
- [ ] Sour cream 2 tbsp
- [ ] Avocado 3 oz
- [ ] Fresh cilantro 1 tsp

PREPARATION

1. Place all ingredients, except for the toppings, into a slow cooker in the order given and stir. Cover and set the slow cooker to high. Cook for about 6 hours, or until the steak is tender.

2. Use a fork to shred some of the steak cubes and break up any tomatoes that remain intact. Serve the chili hot with desired topping.

DINNER

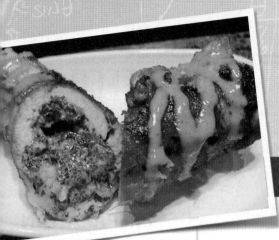

CHICKEN PESTO ROULADE

INGREDIENTS

- [ ] Chicken breasts 4
- [ ] Cheese of choice ¾ cup
- [ ] Pesto 2 oz
- [ ] Olive oil 1 tbsp
- [ ] 1 Lemon Zest
- [ ] Garlic 1 tsp
- [ ] Salt 1 tsp
- [ ] Pepper 1 tsp
- [ ] Olive oil 2 tbsp

PREPARATION

1. Pat your chicken breasts dry of any moisture using paper towels. Cut breasts 1/8" thick, *or pound flat with meat tenderizer.*

2. In a bowl, combine pesto and olive oil. Spread your pesto out on the chicken breasts and zest 1 lemon over the chicken.

3. Chop the cheese into small pieces and spread it out into the chicken. *Roll your chicken up end to end as best as you can.*

4. Tie the chicken together *using either butchers string, or secure it with toothpicks.*

5. Preheat your oven to 450F, and then bring 2 tablespoons olive oil to its smoke point in a cast iron skillet.

6. Add your chicken to the pan and cook it on all sides, *making sure you get a nice sear on the whole outside of the chicken.*

7. Put the pan in the oven for 6-7 minutes to allow the chicken to cook through. *Once the chicken's juices run clear, remove from the oven, let rest for 5-6 minutes, and serve.*

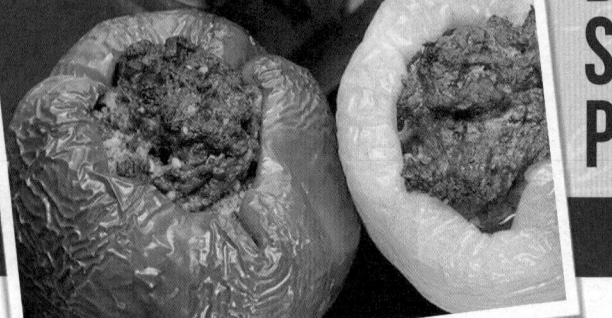

BEEF STUFFED PEPPERS

SERVES: 4 - PREP: 3 HRS.

INGREDIENTS

- [ ] Ground beef 1.5 lb
- [ ] Bacon 4 slices
- [ ] Bell peppers 1 tsp
- [ ] Olive oil 3 tbsp
- [ ] Soy sauce 1 tsp
- [ ] Minced garlic 1 tsp
- [ ] Sugar-free ketchup 1 tsp
- [ ] Oregano 1 tsp
- [ ] Worcestershire 1.5 tsp
- [ ] Hot sauce 1 tsp
- [ ] Liquid smoke 1 tsp
- [ ] Ground black pepper ½ tsp

PREPARATION

1. Put your ground beef inside a Ziploc bag. Add all of the spices to the to the bag, including the oil. Mix all the meat and spices together well *so that everything is thoroughly combined. Let the mixture marinate in the fridge for 3 hours.*

2. Once you are ready to cook, remove the meat mixture from the fridge.

3. Take out the cores of 4 bell peppers. *Be careful with this as you can cut the side of the peppers open and the juice won't stay inside from the meat.*

4. Dice bacon. Fry the bacon until it is partially cooked.

5. Start to boil a pot of water that's heavily salted. Also, preheat your oven to 350F.

6. Add your peppers to the water, *fill them with water so they sink to the bottom.* Boil the peppers for 3 minutes, then remove and drain.

7. While the peppers are cooling, add your bacon and bacon fat to the beef. *Mix everything until combined evenly.*

8. Put your bell peppers onto a foiled tray. Stuff the peppers with the meat mixture *until it's partially coming out of the top.* Then place peppers in oven for 50 minutes.

9. Sprinkle with cheese if desired, then put peppers under the broiler for about 2-3 minutes, *or until the cheese is nicely melted. Cool and serve.*

THE SHEPHERD'S
CODE

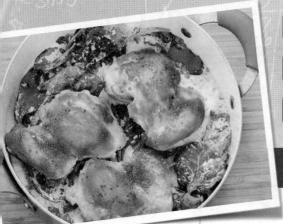

CREAMY CHICKEN GREENS

INGREDIENTS

- [ ] Boneless chicken thighs 1 lb
- [ ] Coconut oil 2 tbsp
- [ ] Chicken stock 1 cup
- [ ] Cream 1 cup
- [ ] Italian herbs 1 tsp
- [ ] Dark leafy greens 16 oz
- [ ] Butter 2 tbsp
- [ ] Coconut flour 2 tbsp
- [ ] Salt and pepper to taste

PREPARATION

1. Preheat a large skillet on medium-high. Add two tablespoons of coconut oil.

2. Season both sides of chicken thighs with salt and pepper, then fry until cooked through and slightly crispy.

3. To prepare the sauce melt two tablespoons of butter in a sauce pan. Once the butter stops sizzling, whisk in two tablespoons of coconut flour to form a thick paste.

4. Whisk in one cup of cream and bring the mixture to a boil. The mixture should thicken after a few minutes. Stir in the teaspoon of Italian herbs.

5. Remove cooked chicken thighs from the skillet and set aside. Pour chicken stock into the chicken skillet and deglaze the pan. Whisk in the cream sauce. Stir the greens into the pan so that they become coated with the sauce.

6. Lay the chicken thighs back on top of the greens, then remove from the heat and serve.

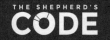

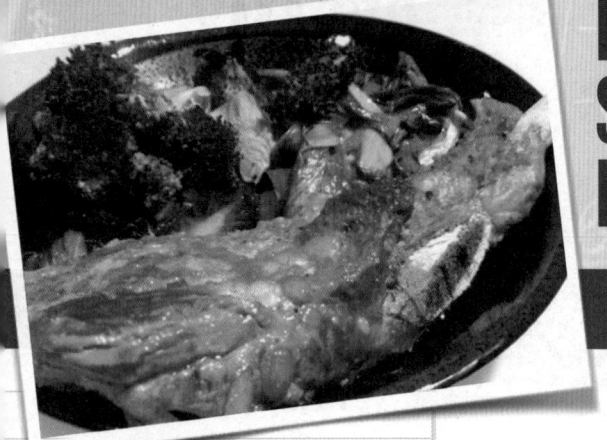

RIBEYE STEAK WITH BROCCOLI

SERVES: 2 - PREP: 30 MINS.

INGREDIENTS

- [ ] 1 Ribeye steak (16 oz)
- [ ] Peanut oil 1 tbsp
- [ ] Butter 1 tbsp
- [ ] Thyme 1/2 tsp
- [ ] Broccoli 4 oz
- [ ] Chestnut paste 2 tbsp
- [ ] Salt and pepper to taste

PREPARATION

1. Preheat the oven to 400F.

2. Rub steak with peanut oil. Sprinkle salt and pepper on all sides to taste.

3. Place cast iron skillet on medium-high heat and sear the steak 2 minutes on each side. Then immediately transfer to oven for 10 minutes.

4. After 10 minutes, take out steak and apply chestnut paste. Add broccoli to skillet and place back to oven and cook for another 10 minutes.

5. After taking out from oven add butter over steak and let it rest for 5 minutes.

6. Serve and enjoy.

THE SHEPHERD'S
CODE

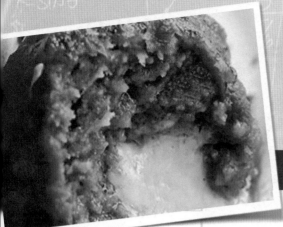

CHEESE FILLED MEATBALLS

SERVES: 4 - TIME: 90 MINS.

INGREDIENTS

Meatball:

- [ ] Ground beef 1 lb
- [ ] Large egg 1 large
- [ ] Garlic 2 cloves
- [ ] Oregano 1 tsp
- [ ] Thyme 1 tsp
- [ ] Coconut flour 1 oz
- [ ] Mozzarella 6 oz
- [ ] Salt and pepper

Topping:

- [ ] Marinara sauce 4 oz
- [ ] Olives 2 oz
- [ ] Fresh coriander for garnish

PREPARATION

1. Preheat your oven to 450F.

2. Dice the mozzarella into 20-25 equal sized pieces. Place them in freezer for 60 minutes (freezing will prevent from leaking out while baking).

3. In a large bowl, add meat, egg, minced garlic, thyme, oregano, coconut flour, salt, pepper and mix until well combined using your hands or a mixer.

4. Divide the meat into 20-25 pieces and flatten each using your hands. Take cheese from the freezer and place 1 piece in the middle of each meatball and fold closed.

5. When all meatballs are assembled, bake for 15 minutes.

6. Heat the marinara sauce in a pan. When meatballs are done, add to the sauce and stir until all are well coated.

7. Garnish with freshly chopped coriander and serve.

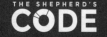

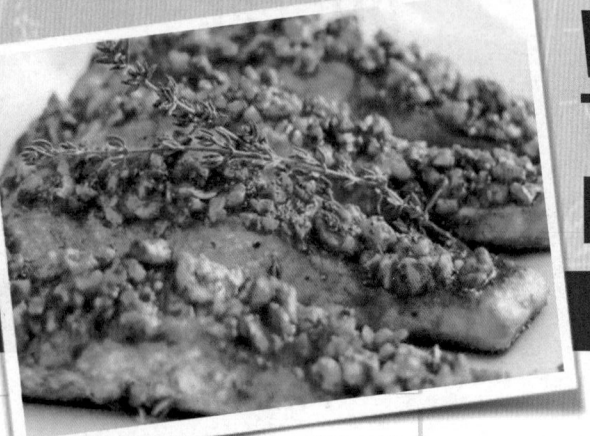

WALNUT TUNA FILET

SERVES: 2 - PREP: 15 MINS.

INGREDIENTS

- [ ] Walnuts 1 oz
- [ ] Raw honey 1 tbsp
- [ ] Mustard ½ tsp
- [ ] Dill ½ tsp
- [ ] Tuna fillets 1.2 lb
- [ ] Olive oil 1 tbsp
- [ ] Salt and pepper to taste
- [ ] Fresh baby kale to taste
- [ ] Smoked paprika to taste

PREPARATION

1. Preheat the oven to 350F.

2. Add walnuts, raw honey, spices, and mustard in a food processor and make a paste.

3. Heat a pan with olive oil and cook dry tuna filets for about 3 minutes, just enough to create a crispy outer texture.

4. Add the walnut paste to the top of the tuna fillets, then transfer to the oven and bake for about 10 minutes.

5. Serve with a little fresh baby kale and smoked paprika. Enjoy!

THE SHEPHERD'S
CODE

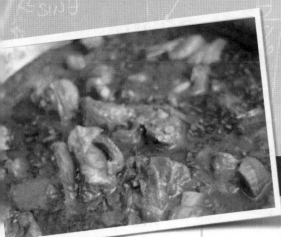

SPICY LAMB STEW

SERVES: 5 - PREP: 45 MINS.

PREPARATION

1. Cut the lamb into small pieces and season with salt, ground pepper, and ginger.

2. Add tomatoes and tomato paste and mix well. Finally add coconut milk and mix again.

3. Cook for 40 minutes on medium heat. After 25 minutes add cream and mix thoroughly.

4. Serve and enjoy.

INGREDIENTS

- [ ] Boneless lamb 1.2 lb
- [ ] Coconut oil 1 fl oz
- [ ] Onion powder 5 tsp
- [ ] Crushed garlic 3 cloves
- [ ] Ginger powder 1 tsp
- [ ] Tomato paste 1.5 oz
- [ ] Garam masala 4 tsp
- [ ] Paprika 1 ½ tsp
- [ ] Salt to taste
- [ ] Diced tomatoes 1 cup
- [ ] Cream ½ cup
- [ ] Coconut milk 1 cup
- [ ] Chopped parsley 1 ½ tbsp

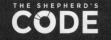

GOUDA STUFFED CHICKEN

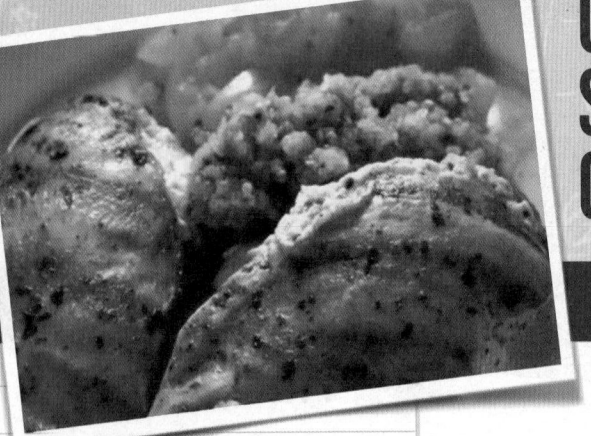

SERVES: 1 - PREP: 20 MINS.

INGREDIENTS

- ☐ 1 boneless skinless chicken breasts ~8 oz
- ☐ Spinach 1 cup
- ☐ Ricotta cheese 2 Tbsp
- ☐ Shredded smoked gouda cheese 1 oz
- ☐ Olive oil 3 Tbsp
- ☐ salt and pepper to taste

PREPARATION

1. Preheat oven to 375F.

2. Put a pan on medium heat and sauté the spinach in butter until it begins to wilt.

3. Butterfly the chicken breast (lay the chicken flat on your cutting board and cut it horizontally, but not all the way through, so you can open it like a book).

4. Use a meat tenderizer to pound the chicken breast flat.

5. Spread the spinach on the inside of the chicken breast, top with cheese, and fold the chicken closed.

6. Bake in the oven for 35 minutes or until chicken is cooked through.

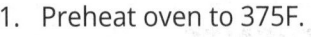

THE SHEPHERD'S
CODE

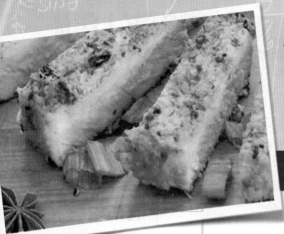

ASIAN INSPIRED PORK CHOPS

SERVES: 4 - PREP: 10 MINS.

INGREDIENTS

- [ ] Boneless pork chops 4
- [ ] Stalk lemongrass (peeled and diced) 2
- [ ] Halved garlic 8 cloves
- [ ] Fish sauce 2 tbsp
- [ ] Almond flour 2 tbsp
- [ ] Soy sauce 3 tsp
- [ ] Sesame oil 2 tsp
- [ ] Five spice 1 tsp
- [ ] Peppercorns 1 tsp

PREPARATION

1. Mix everything except the pork chops and almond flour to create a marinade. Mix well in a large bowl.

2. Dunk the pork chops in the marinade bowl (or let them soak in the refrigerator for 2 hours beforehand if you have time).

3. Dredge pork chops in almond flour to a bowl. The marinade will help the flour stick and form a kind of breading.

4. Cook the pork chops in a pan greased with ghee for 4-5 minutes on each side.

5. Cut into strips and serve.

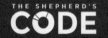

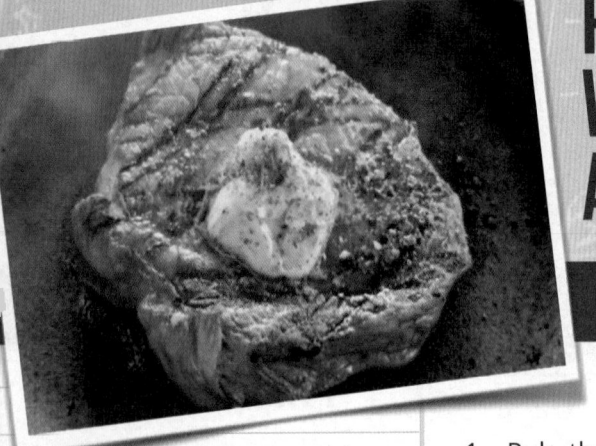

PORK LOIN WITH AVOCADO

SERVES: 1 - PREP: 15 MINS.

INGREDIENTS

- [ ] Pork loin 1
- [ ] Butter 1 Tbsp
- [ ] Yellow mustard 1 tsp
- [ ] Salt and pepper to taste

Ingredients for sauce:

- [ ] Avocado ½
- [ ] Garlic 1 clove
- [ ] juice of ½ a lemon
- [ ] Mayo 2 Tbsp

PREPARATION

1. Rub the pork with mustard and season with salt and pepper.

2. Melt the butter in a pan on medium heat, then cook the pork loin for 5-8 minutes. Flip and cook again on the other side.

3. Transfer to a serving plate.

4. Add the sauce ingredients to a blender. Blend, then drizzle over the pork loin.

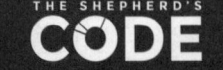

THE SHEPHERD'S CODE

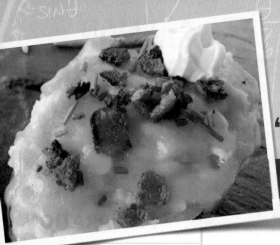

CAULI-FLOWER "BAKED POTATO"

SERVES: 2 - PREP: 25 MINS.

INGREDIENTS

- ☐ Chopped cauliflower 1 head
- ☐ Large ripe avocado 1
- ☐ Sea salt 1 tsp
- ☐ Cracked black pepper ¼ tsp
- ☐ Heavy cream 1 tbsp
- ☐ Butter 4 tbsp
- ☐ Onion powder ½ tsp
- ☐ Shredded cheddar 2 oz
- ☐ Crumbled bacon 2 oz
- ☐ Green onions 1 tbsp
- ☐ Chopped chives 1 tsp
- ☐ Sour cream 1 tsp
- ☐ Blue cheese 2 tbsp

PREPARATION

1. Preheat your oven to 375F.

2. Steam the cauliflower for about 10 minutes, or until fork-tender.

3. Meanwhile, cook bacon until crisp, then crumble. Also slice the avocado and melt the butter.

4. Using a blender, combine steamed cauliflower, butter, avocado, salt, pepper, cream, and onion. Blend until it smooth.

5. Add green onions, bacon (try to save some for the topping) and blend until smooth. Spoon this mixture into the avocado shells.

6. Top with cheddar cheese and blue cheese. Bake for 15 minutes. Remove and top with crumbled bacon, chives, and sour cream.

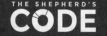

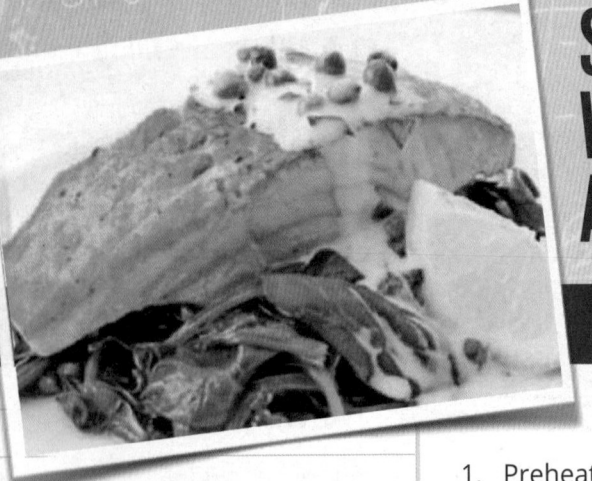

SALMON WITH SPIN- ACH SAUCE

SERVES: 1 - TIME: 30 MINS.

PREPARATION

1. Preheat your oven to 400F

2. Wash salmon and place on a baking tray. Season to taste and brush with ghee. Bake for 25 minutes.

3. Meanwhile, heat a skillet on medium heat. Grease with ghee and cook spinach for 5 minutes.

4. Now, add whipping cream (or coconut milk) and set aside.

5. On a serving plate place baked salmon on a bed of creamed spinach, pour hollandaise sauce on top.

INGREDIENTS

- ☐ Salmon 7 oz
- ☐ Spinach 5 oz
- ☐ Heavy whipping cream 1 tbsp
- ☐ Ghee 2 tbsp
- ☐ Hollandaise sauce
- ☐ Salt and pepper to taste

THE SHEPHERD'S
CODE

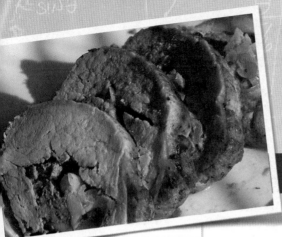

TRIPLE PORK ROAST

SERVES: 6 - TIME: 70 MINS.

PREPARATION

1. Preheat oven to 375F.

2. Cut the tenderloin lengthwise almost all the way through leaving out about ½ inch so you can then open the tenderloin like a book.

3. Cook ground sausage, diced onions, and minced garlic in ghee until browned- approx. 10 minutes. When done, transfer to a mixing bowl. Add sage and flax meal and season with salt and pepper to taste. Toss and set aside.

4. Place the sausage stuffing inside the tenderloin and roll up tightly. Wrap the tenderloin in bacon strips, securing with toothpicks if necessary.

5. Place the tenderloin on a baking sheet and bake for 45 minutes. Remove and let it rest for 15 minutes before slicing and serving.

6. Remove the toothpicks and serve.

INGREDIENTS

- ☐ Pork tenderloin 1 lb
- ☐ Ghee 1 tbsp
- ☐ Red onion 2 oz
- ☐ Garlic 2 cloves
- ☐ Ground sausage 14 oz
- ☐ Thyme 1 tsp
- ☐ Bacon 8 oz
- ☐ Salt and pepper to taste

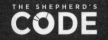

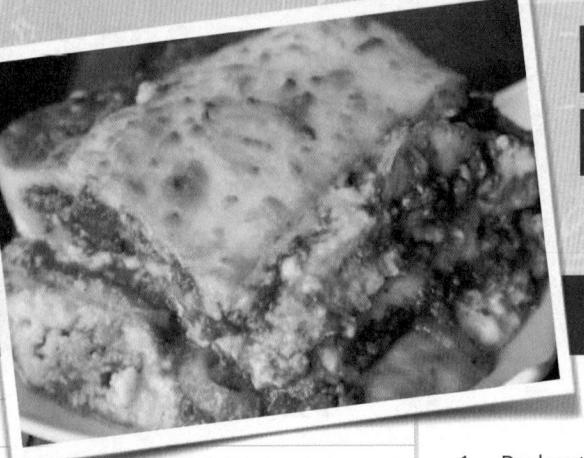

KETO LASAGNA

INGREDIENTS

- [ ] Eggplant 1.5 lb
- [ ] Marinara sauce 10 oz
- [ ] Fresh baby spinach 10 oz
- [ ] Feta cheese 7 oz
- [ ] Mozzarella cheese 4 oz
- [ ] Parmesan cheese 1 oz
- [ ] Eggs 6
- [ ] Ghee 3 oz
- [ ] Salt and pepper to taste

PREPARATION

1. Preheat your oven to 400F.

2. Slice eggplant into ½ inch slices and place on a baking tray. Brush with ghee, sprinkle with salt, and bake for 20 minutes. When done, set aside and reduce oven to 360F.

3. Meanwhile wilt spinach in a pan with ghee.

4. Make 6 thin "omelets" by whisking an egg, pouring it into the hot pan, and swirling until the egg makes a wide circle. When edges begin to pull up, flip and cook the other side. Repeat until you have 6 omelets.

5. Start assembling the lasagna by laying down a row of eggplant, a layer of omelet, then spinach, cheese, and marinara. Alternate until all ingredients are used up.

6. Bake for 30 minutes or until top looks crispy and golden brown. Let cool before serving.

BEEF SHORT-RIB CURRY

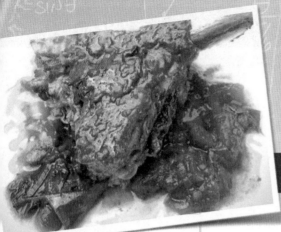

SERVES: 4 - PREP: 6 HRS.

INGREDIENTS

- [ ] Beef ribs 2 lb (8 pieces)
- [ ] Coconut oil 1 fl oz
- [ ] Ghee 2 tbsp
- [ ] Salt and pepper to taste
- [ ] White wine ½ cup
- [ ] Fresh tomato sauce ¾ cup
- [ ] Fresh tomatoes 1 cup
- [ ] Freshly chopped garlic cloves 3
- [ ] Chopped rainbow chard leaves 6 oz
- [ ] Chopped celery stalks 4 oz

PREPARATION

1. Take 8 beef ribs and season with freshly cracked pepper and a few pinches of salt.

2. Add coconut oil or ghee to a hot pan. Sear the ribs until browned on all sides, then transfer to a crockpot.

3. Add white wine to the pan.

4. Add Marsala to the pan and deglaze. Add tomatoes and tomato sauce to the pan, stirring occasionally.

5. Pour everything from the pan over the ribs in the crockpot, then add remaining ingredients to crockpot. Mix well so that some vegetables are on top and some are on the bottom.

6. Cook on high for 6 hours. Do not lift the lid except maybe once to turn the ribs over.

7. Serve with cauliflower rice or zucchini noodles.

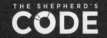

BONUS: DESSERTS

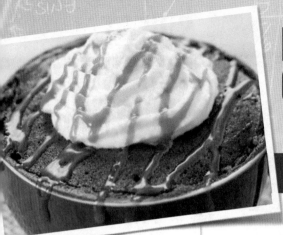

MOCHA CAKE

SERVES: 1 - PREP: 5 MINS.

PREPARATION

1. Combine all dry ingredients in a mug and mix thoroughly.

2. Add the egg, ghee, erythritol, and mix well with a fork.

3. Microwave for 90 seconds.

4. Top with whipped cream and serve in the mug.

INGREDIENTS

- ☐ Almond flour 2 tbsp
- ☐ Egg 1
- ☐ Raw cocoa powder 1 tbsp
- ☐ Mocha powder 1 tbsp
- ☐ Baking soda 1 tsp
- ☐ Erythritol 2 tbsp
- ☐ Ghee 1 tbsp
- ☐ Whipped cream 2 tbsp

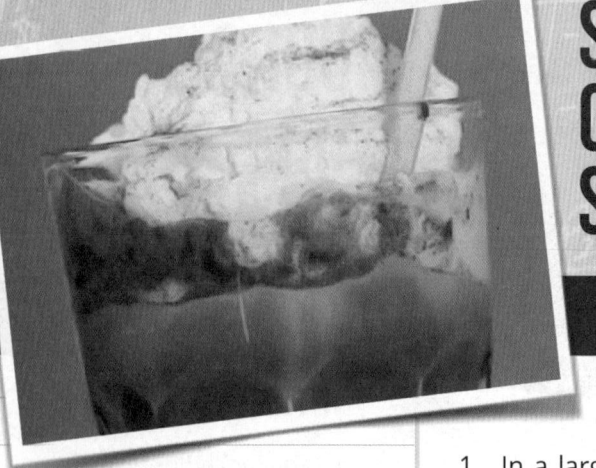

SWEET COCONUT SMOOTHIE

SERVES: 1 - PREP: 5 MINS.

INGREDIENTS

- [ ] Unsweetened coconut milk 2 cups
- [ ] Cappuccino coffee 2 tsp
- [ ] Cocoa powder 1 tsp
- [ ] Coconut extract ½ tsp
- [ ] Stevia 5/6 fl oz
- [ ] Protein powder 1 tsp

PREPARATION

1. In a large cup, add all your ingredients together. Stir well, do not worry if everything does not integrate well.

2. Place in a flat, freezer safe bowl. Every few hours, scratch the mixture with a fork.

3. After it's frozen and once ready to serve, leave it on the counter until it softens.

4. Put it in a blender or food processor and mix thoroughly. Serve and enjoy!

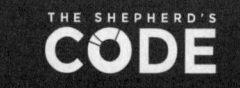

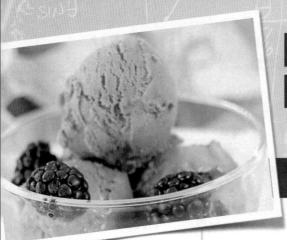

BLACKBERRY ICE CREAM

SERVES: 6 - PREP: 330 MINS.

PREPARATION

1. Place a pan over medium-low heat and add heavy cream and erythritol. Don't boil it, just wait until erythritol is dissolved slightly.

2. Meanwhile, add egg yolks in a mixing bowl and beat using hand mixer until they've doubled in size.

3. Now, add hot cream mixture gently into the egg mixture and mix. Add berry extract, protein powder, and xanthan gum and mix well.

4. Place the bowl in the freezer for 2 hours minimum, occasionally taking out to stir.

5. Meanwhile, put black berries in a mixer (it should be little chunky). When the ice cream looks a bit thicker, it's the right time to add the chunky black berries and mix gently, but don't over mix.

6. Let this ice cream chill for another 4 hours or overnight before tasting.

INGREDIENTS

- ☐ Heavy cream 8 oz
- ☐ Erythritol 2 oz
- ☐ Blackberries 6 oz
- ☐ Vanilla protein powder 2 oz
- ☐ Large egg yolks 3
- ☐ Berry extract ½ tsp
- ☐ Xanthan gum 1/8 tsp

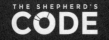

YUMMY BROWNIES

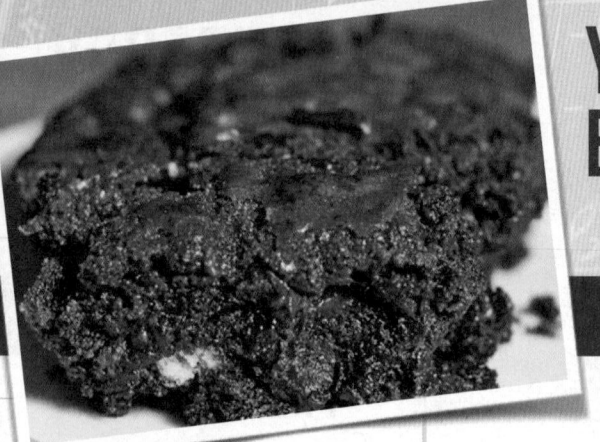

SERVES: 8 - PREP: 35 MINS.

PREPARATION

1. Preheat oven to 350F.

2. Add caramel to a bowl and mix well.

3. In a separate bowl, combine the almond flour, cocoa powder, baking soda, and salt. Then combine the two bowls and mix them thoroughly with a hand mixer.

4. Put the dough into a baking dish and bake for 25 minutes. Let the brownies cool for 5 minutes and cut them into 8 equal parts then serve.

INGREDIENTS

- ☐ Almond flour 2 cups
- ☐ Cocoa powder ½ cup
- ☐ Sweetener 1 ½ tbsp
- ☐ Coconut oil 2 fl oz
- ☐ Honey 1 oz
- ☐ Eggs 2
- ☐ Caramel 2 tsp
- ☐ Baking soda ½ tsp
- ☐ Salt to taste

CELLULAR REJUVENATION SECRETS MANUAL

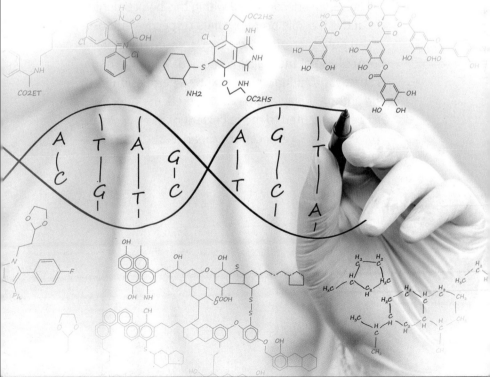

THE SHEPHERD'S
CODE

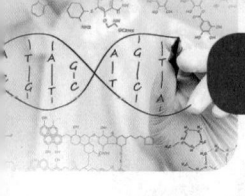

The contents of this document are based upon my opinions of *The Shepherd's Code* unless otherwise noted. This work is intended to share knowledge and information learned through research, experience, and discussions with others. The opinions of others, such as in the comments and the forum, are their own and are not endorsed by *The Shepherd's Code*. The information contained herein is not intended to diagnose, treat, cure or prevent any condition or disease, but rather to provide general information that is intended to be used for educational purposes only. Please consult with your physician or healthcare practitioner if you have any concerns. By using, viewing and interacting with *The Shepherd's Code* or **shepherdscode.com** website, you agree to all terms of engagement, thus assuming complete responsibility for your own actions. The authors and publishers will not claim accountability, nor shall they be held liable for any loss or injury sustained by you. Use, view and interact with these resources at your own risk. All products and information given to you by *The Shepherd's Code* and its related companies are strictly for informational purposes only. While every attempt has been made to verify the accuracy of information provided on our website and within our publications, neither the authors nor the publishers are responsible for assuming liability for possible inaccuracies. The authors and publishers disclaim any responsibility for the inaccuracy of the content, including but not limited to errors or omissions. Loss of property, injury to self or others, and even death could occur as a direct or indirect consequence of the use and application of any content found herein. Please act responsibly. The information provided may need to be downloaded and/or viewed using third party software, such as Acrobat. It's the user's responsibility to install the software necessary to view such information. Any downloads, whether purchased or given for free from our website, related websites or hosting systems are performed at the user's own risk. Although we take great preventative measures, we cannot warranty that our websites are free of corrupting computer codes, viruses or worms. If you are a minor, you can use this service only with permission and guidance from your parents or guardians.

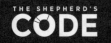

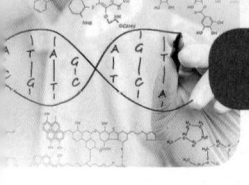
Peace I leave with you; my peace I give to you. Not as the world gives do I give to you. Let not your hearts be troubled, neither let them be afraid.

John 14:27

Stress. Who needs it? Jesus knew we needed some assurance in this area. He gave us his peace but we have a hard time holding onto it at times. I think many would agree that much of our day is spent dealing with stress while doing our best to avoid more of it. We do our chores so that the stress of piled up laundry isn't hanging over our heads. We go to work to earn money so as to avoid the stress of bills.

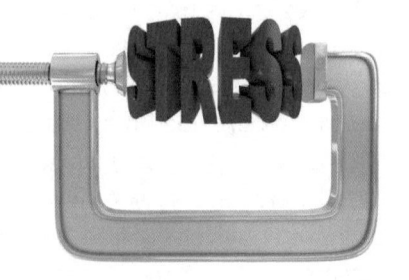

But look and listen; you will find that lurking just beneath the surface of our skin is a different type of stress that has been calling out for our attention. It goes by the name of **oxidative stress.** And in case you didn't know, stress is cumulative! **It builds and builds and builds until we do something to mitigate it.**

Signs of oxidative stress wreaking havoc in our body result from the blended effect of oxygen we breathe combined with byproducts created as cells metabolize this oxygen into energy. At any one time within our bodies, oxidation is occurring through millions of normal natural processes.

For example, as the immune system fights off infection, it creates **inflammation and oxidation** takes place. Oxidation also occurs as the liver and kidneys detoxify the myriad contaminates we've ingested by eating and breathing each day. Chemical additives, refined sugars, and highly processed foods are just some of the digested toxins that our bodies become overwhelmed with as they are broken down and metabolized. Furthermore, physical and emotional stresses significantly increase the oxidation process as well.

Would you believe that even **exercise can cause oxidative stress**? This is why movement is important but killing ourselves at the gym is counterintuitive. Thirty minutes, four times per week is adequate time

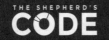

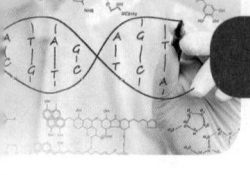
for exercise. I remember a few years ago when I received my CrossFit Certification, I was so excited! I would spend hours at the gym doing 100 pull-ups, 100 sit-ups, 100 squats and then run a mile! This was my 'normal' for years.

Well, one day I decided to take the day off from the gym. I felt so amazing the following morning, I was stunned. I started researching exercise and stress on the body. Sure enough, over doing it in the gym saps the body of important hormones and can be detrimental. **Moderate exercise is much healthier and beneficial.** I soon stopped trying to be Wonder Woman.

WHAT'S THE BIG DEAL?

Oxidation is what happens to a sliced apple as it sits out and turns brown, or an old broken-down truck is left exposed to the elements over time and develops rust. Yuck! **Who wants rusty mushy insides?**

But wait, there's more. As cells begin to oxidize they deteriorate and affect further damage by releasing byproducts called free radicals into the body. Free radicals are unstable molecules that damage cells or create abnormal ones, even attacking our DNA.

This natural release of free radicals within our body is balanced by another automatic response initiated to repair these damaged cells. When this balance is overwhelmed by too many free radicals the **repair process becomes insufficient and can't combat the harmful molecules**.

 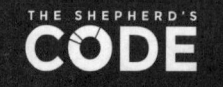

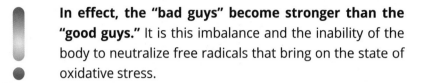

In effect, the "bad guys" become stronger than the "good guys." It is this imbalance and the inability of the body to neutralize free radicals that bring on the state of oxidative stress.

WHY IS THIS HARMFUL?

Oxidative Stress greatly impedes the body's ability to perform at its best. Left unchecked, this stress leads to disease and significant disruption of important bodily functions. Free radicals resulting from oxidation have been linked to what we typically consider as signs of aging.

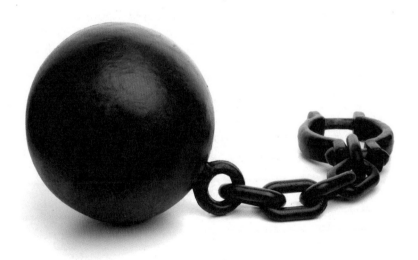

Remember also your Creator in the days of
your youth, before the evil days come and the
years draw near of which you will say, "I have
no pleasure in them"; before the sun and the
light and the moon and the stars are darkened
and the clouds return after the rain, in the
day when the keepers of the house tremble,
and the strong men are bent, and the grinders
cease because they are few, and those who
look through the windows are dimmed, and
the doors on the street are shut—when the
sound of the grinding is low, and one rises up
at the sound of a bird, and all the daughters
of song are brought low—they are afraid also
of what is high, and terrors are in the way; the
almond tree blossoms, the grasshopper drags
itself along, and desire fails, because man is
going to his eternal home, and the mourners
go about the streets— ...

Ecclesiastes 12:1-14

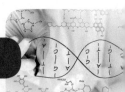
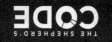

This poetic description of aging can seem so sad. I wish we could say things are different now. But it seems to me that plenty of people are aging just this way still today. Many of the symptoms could point towards oxidative stress left unchecked. It's so harmful that it hastens the aging process and also causes a number of neurodegenerative diseases and also a few cardiovascular diseases.

A few such diseases are:

- **Hyperoxia**
- **Irradiation**
- **Tissue injury**
- **Neurodegenerative Diseases**

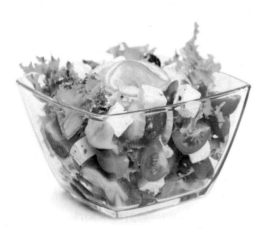

Deficiency in our nutrition also has a role to play in oxidative stress. The habit of eating junk food and fast food is one reason we end up nutrient deficient. Such foods deprive our body of vitamins and minerals. In this case, your best option is to turn toward a **diet that is rich in vitamins, minerals and fiber.**

From the outside in, we experience the attacks of oxidative stress in so many ways.

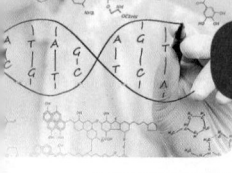
These are just some of the signs that oxidative stress may be winning the battle in your body:

- gray hair
- joint pain
- fatigue
- wrinkles
- memory loss

- headaches
- diseases, even cancer
- weakened immune system

HOW LOW-FAT DIETS INCREASE OXIDATIVE STRESS

Amanda Holliday, MS, RD, LDN, a clinical associate professor in the Department of Nutrition at the University of North Carolina at Chapel Hill, said that eating fat plays an important role in maintaining good health. Eating fats also makes you feel satiety or fullness, **she said:**

"We don't feel quite as hungry, and that may help with weight control."

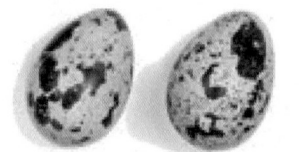

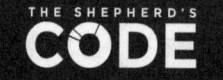

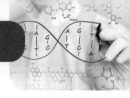

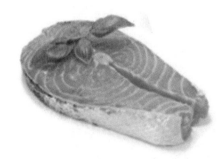

From personal experience, not feeling 'quite as hungry' is an understatement! The lack of hunger keeps your mind and body focused on the task at hand. There is no more thinking about dinner while eating lunch! Food addiction disappears when eating this high fat, moderate protein, low carb food plan. It truly is a lifestyle, not just a diet!

When I went away to college, I developed an eating disorder called bulimia/anorexia. I starved, over exercised and binged and purged occasionally. I was a mess. I remember I ate the same thing everyday (without variation). **Breakfast was coffee, Lunch was an apple and half a ham and cheese sandwich and dinner a small salad.** I got down to 114 lbs.! At almost 5'9, this is ridiculously thin! I thought I was fat! This disease is insidious, baffling and cunning! I needed help.

When I went home for the holidays, my family was astounded by my appearance. My mother plainly said, "Get help, or we won't pay your college tuition." So, I got help! I went to rehab for thirty five days in Orlando, Fl.! In rehab I learned that sugar, wheat and flour can cause a phenomenon of craving for more and more sugar! These items were removed from my food plan! No sugar, wheat or flour ever! I stuck to this for many, many years. The adjustment I had to make was to substitute high fat (nuts, olive oil, coconut oil, cheese) for carbs like potatoes, bananas and rice. Anytime I ate a carb, I felt awful! I stopped eating them! The cravings disappeared and so did my eating disorder! **It was truly miraculous! This plan worked!**

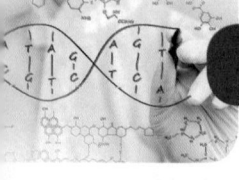
The irony was, I gained enough weight to look human but I was still super lean because that's what *The Shepherd's Code System* does!

The afflicted shall eat and be satisfied; those who seek him shall praise the Lord! May your hearts live forever!

Psalm 22:26

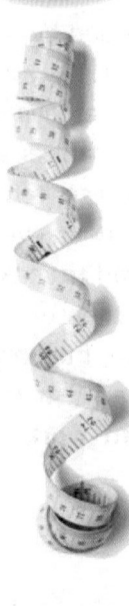

Regardless of these facts, nutritionists began to advocate a low-fat diet decades ago. They recommended that consumers replace fat in their diets with healthier foods. What followed was that **many companies started offering packaged foods that were low in fat but high in sugar and refined flour.** We know now that what took the place of the fats are the exact things that cause an increase in our oxidative stress. "The companies were really playing up the fact they were in low in fat when in fact that didn't make them a healthy choice at all," Hobbs said.

In the midst of this advertising blitz, many "health conscious" consumers overlooked **what was key in that message.** They ignored that achieving a healthy diet meant reducing their consumption of sweets, refined carbohydrates, saturated and trans fats while increasing the intake of fruits, vegetables, and whole grains. Ignoring the parts of a diet that would take some effort left millions in danger of worsening rather than improving their health.

> *He shall eat curds and honey when he knows how to refuse the evil and choose the good.*
>
> **Isaiah 7:15**

Also, **extreme exercise**, like marathon training, CrossFit and hot yoga (if done too frequently), can cause oxidative stress. It is NOT necessary to kill yourself in the gym! Breathing, moving and an elevated heart rate in the fat burning zone (depending one one's age, it varies) is the best way to exercise.

Alas, there is hope...

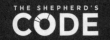

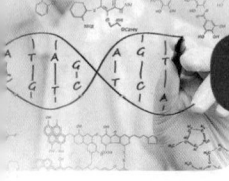
CAN I PROTECT MYSELF FROM OXIDATIVE STRESS?

Now that you know **some of the causes** of oxidative stress on your body, you are able to make informed choices that will decrease and avoid the negative effects. One angle you can suit up for will fight this battle externally. Another option is closer to home and attacks the culprits from the inside.

> This external strategy altogether avoids exposure to the harmful causes of oxidation. For many of us, that might mean we would need to move inside a bubble to shield ourselves from things such as pollution, or contaminated air and water. More realistically, using **household products** free of dyes, chemicals, and toxins is a more tangible option.

Conversely, a battle fought from the inside initially requires introducing a host of antioxidants, foods that will reverse the damage caused by **free radicals** on the loose in your body. Antioxidants are like the soldiers/medics that can get up close to the affected cells, destroy the bad guys, heal what has been damaged, and provide protection for the rest. There is a solid plan that puts these measures into practice. It is a way for us to best feed and care for our body. It is called *The Shepherd's Code System.*

As I mentioned above, oxidative stress becomes a reality for those of us with a diet high in **refined sugars**, chemicals, and processed foods. To reduce oxidative stress a specific diet utilizing powerful foods rich in antioxidants and "healing fats" is essential. The more frequently we can replace these toxins with organic and healthy, nutrient rich foods, the better. This is great news. **This is the solution!**

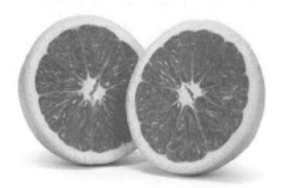

Scientists at Gladstone Institutes support the findings that the low-carb, low-calorie diet has an anti-aging effect found to **protect cells** from oxidative stress. This diet is the winning recipe that actually reduces exposure to contaminants as well as regains the **body's healthy balance**.

For millions of years, our species followed a high "healing fats" diet. This diet was an **essential part of the lifestyle** in which our brains developed and evolved. Alarmingly, with a change in diet and lifestyle we have seen that the human brain is not only shrinking but with age brain atrophy has begun to seem normal.

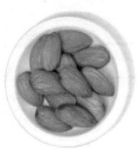

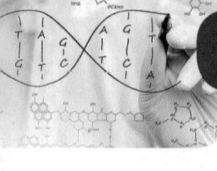

Our bodies have become **less efficient** at removing the free radicals leaving us with a toxic overload of oxidative stress. This health crisis drives our call to action: We must be increasingly vigilant about feeding ourselves the foods that will fight the stresses that damage our very cells and DNA.

HOW DOES THE SHEPHERD'S CODE SYSTEM WORK?

A person following *The Shepherd's Code System* derives their healing source of energy from **ketones** that come from the normal metabolism of fat.

The body is able to use this energy in a safer and more effective way than the energy we get from eating carbohydrates, or sugar. Our organs function more effectively and efficiently when fat derived ketones are their source of fuel. The fuel we pump into our body is what powers the brain, heart, and primary detox center—the kidneys, to name

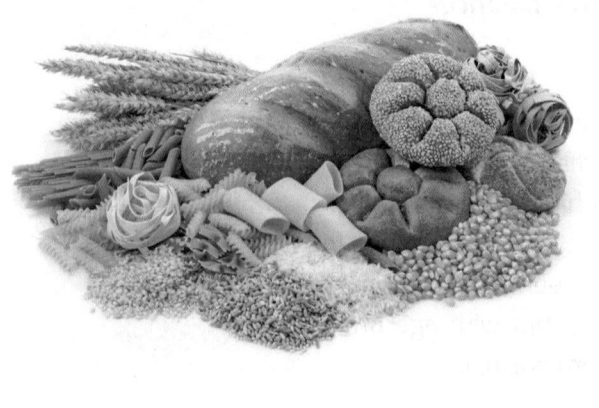

just a few. What we put in is what we get out. We simply **can't afford** to skimp on our fuel sources.

As Christian B. Allan, Ph.D. and Wolfgang Lutz, MD said in their book Life Without Bread: "**Carbohydrates are not required to obtain energy.**

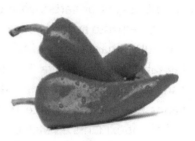

Fat supplies more energy than a comparable amount of carbohydrate, and low-carbohydrate diets tend to make your system of producing energy more efficient. Furthermore, many organs prefer fat for energy." So, **don't fear fat**, instead embrace "healing fats"!

HOW DO I USE THE SHEPHERD'S CODE SYSTEM TO REDUCE OXIDATIVE STRESS?

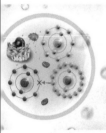

> Here's how you can slow and possibly stop oxidative stress:

▶ STEP 1

Significantly reduce carbohydrates in your diet... Fewer than 20 grams per day is a great place to start.

▶ STEP 2

Set the body into a state of ketosis. In ketosis, we use our own body fat for energy. You become a machine that burns fat all day rather than

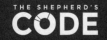

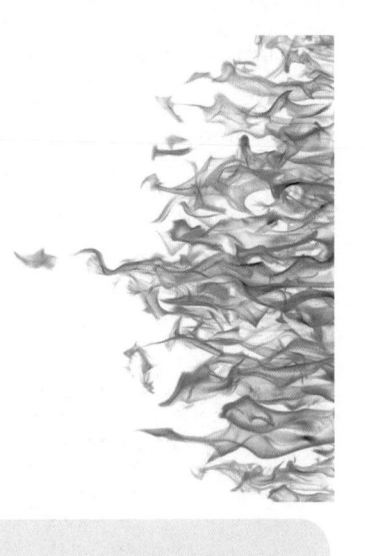

simple sugars or carbohydrates. We set this system into action by making healthy fats our primary supply of calories. "Healing fats" include omega 3s found in oily fish, and walnuts, among others. Avocados are another source that is chock full of antioxidants as well. Incorporating these as a replacement for foods high in carbohydrates is one solid step on the way to reducing oxidative stress.

▶ STEP 3

Seek quality over quantity. For those particularly seeking the fountain of youth it is advisable to look for foods of high nutritional and antioxidant value. Organic foods are ideal. These are free of the pesticides and toxins that cause damage in the first place.

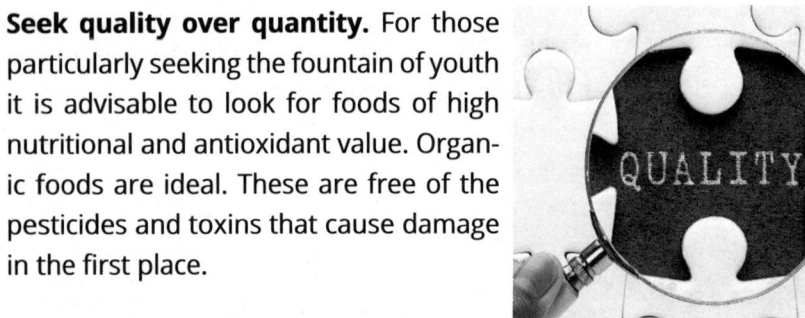

Keep in mind that antioxidant-rich foods will attack free radicals and eliminate the oxidative stress that ages skin, hair, eyes, and even the brain. Consider drinking green tea as an excellent source of antioxidants. It is known to have weight-loss benefits as well.

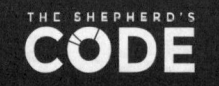

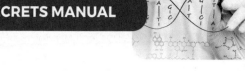

WHAT ARE THE BENEFITS OF THE SHEPHERD'S CODE SYSTEM?

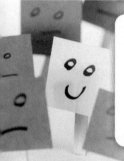

A **low-carb diet** that is rich in "healing fats" has innumerable positive effects on an individual. According to Kris Gunners BSc, these are just some of the ways a high fat diet can change lives for the better:

Decreased hunger—People who cut carbs and substitute healthy fats and proteins end up consuming fewer calories because they feel fuller longer and have sustained energy from the food they eat.

People on low-carb high "healing fat" diets tend to lose **more weight** than others. Low-carb diets result in the body shedding excess water as insulin levels become balanced.

Much of the fat burned from a high fat diet is from the **abdominal cavity**. Visceral fat is what surrounds the organs of the abdominal cavity and leads to metabolic dysfunction.

Lower **triglycerides**—Triglycerides are fat molecules in the blood that are a known risk factor for heart disease.

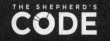

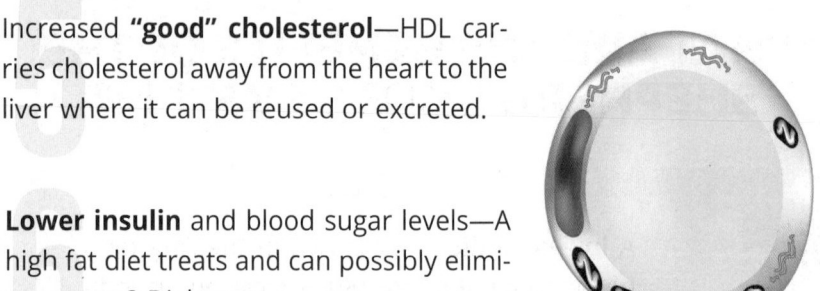

Increased **"good" cholesterol**—HDL carries cholesterol away from the heart to the liver where it can be reused or excreted.

Lower insulin and blood sugar levels—A high fat diet treats and can possibly eliminate type 2 Diabetes.

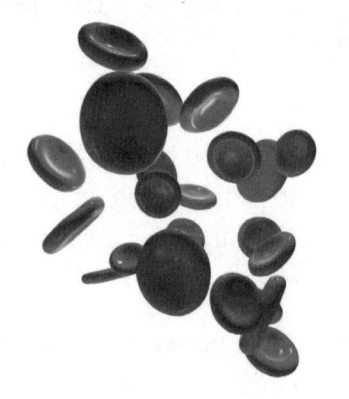

Lower blood pressure or hypertension—This reduces the risk for many serious diseases caused by hypertension.

The Shepherd's Code System has the potential to reverse all 5 symptoms of **metabolic syndrome**. Metabolic syndrome predisposes someone to heart disease and type 2 diabetes.

The Shepherd's Code System is therapeutic for **several brain disorders**. Studies continue for the benefits of the a high fat diet to treat Alzheimer's, Epilepsy, and Parkinson's.

It is wonderful to note that **for so many of the ailments** that plague our loved ones, ourselves, and those who have passed, there continue to be advancements in technology and wisdom for the way we live.

 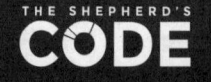

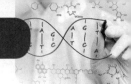

HOW DO I BEGIN?

If any of you lacks wisdom, let him ask God, who gives generously to all without reproach, and it will be given him.

James 1:5

Congratulations, you already have begun. Suit up with the faith that you have God's power at your request. You also have the support of others learning and sharing this journey alongside you. Educating yourself on the benefits of a high fat diet arms you with the knowledge you need to enact change. When you know better, you do better.

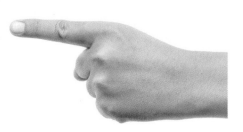

It's true that a functional high fat diet takes **vigilance**, **commitment** and **desire**. A focused plan of action is important. Buying the appropriate foods and having guidance, following the plan are great ways to start.

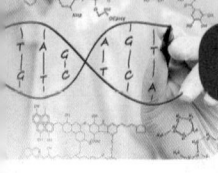
WHERE DO I GO FROM HERE?

Follow the suggestions I have for you and return again to learn more, if you find that temptation is an issue make sure to stay active in the *The Shepherd's Code Facebook group* by going here **www.shepcodefamily.com**.

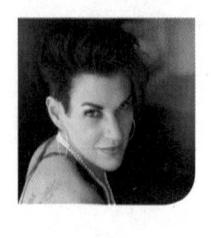

All things are possible!

Kristina Wilds

ANTI-ANXIETY & STRESS ELIMINATION GUIDE

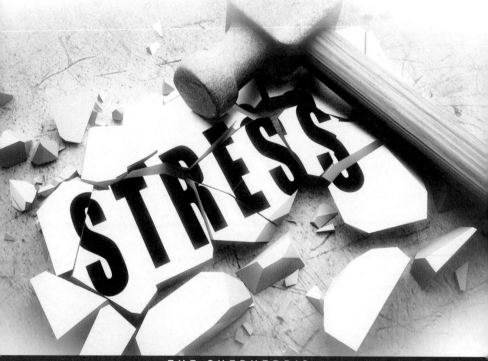

THE SHEPHERD'S CODE

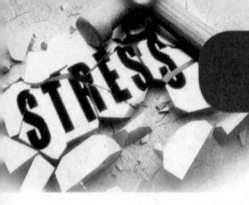

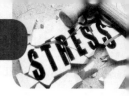

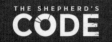

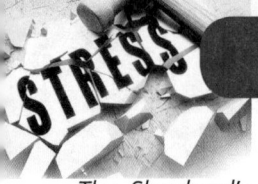

The Shepherd's Code isn't just about losing weight... It's certainly one of the biggest benefits of switching your body from burning sugar to burning fat, but there are many more positive changes you will see.

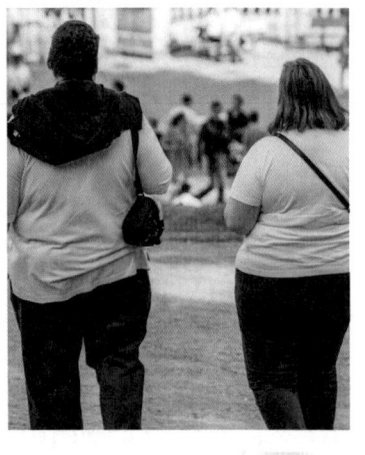

One way to ensure you live a healthy and long life is to understand and manage anxiety and stress. We can choose a heavenly perspective to keep the importance of "the little things" in check.

"Therefore I tell you, do not be anxious about your life, what you will eat or what you will drink, nor about your body, what you will put on. Is not life more than food, and the body more than clothing? Look at the birds of the air: they neither sow nor reap nor gather into barns, and yet your heavenly Father feeds them. Are you not of more value than they? And which of you by being anxious can add a single hour to his span of life? And why are you anxious about clothing? Consider the lilies of the field, how they grow: they neither toil nor spin, yet I tell you, even Solomon in all his glory was not arrayed like one of these. ...

Matthew 6:25-34

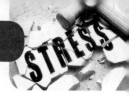

Every year, more than 600,000 people die in the US from heart-related problems. In 2017, it is estimated that over 1.5 million people will have been diagnosed with cancer in the States. These depressing, terrible numbers aren't any more uplifting for lung ailments, suicides, liver cirrhosis, and accidents.

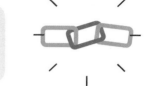

The connecting link between these seemingly unrelated causes: **Stress.**

More and more people throughout the world are experiencing depression and anxiety, and our fast-paced lives can often make us feel like we're suffocating. Pressure that we feel everywhere, from our peers (both virtual and in real life), our bosses, our families, and our finances, is rising and there is seemingly nothing we can do about it.

But there's good news: We can change the way we are dealing with these situations.

In this bonus report, we will define stress, and explain how it leads to anxiety, affects your health, and impacts your diet. I'll then show you several simple and actionable ways to relieve some or all of it.

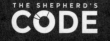

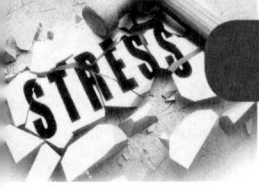
STRESS AND ITS EFFECT ON OUR MENTAL HEALTH

Stress is a term that we often use casually without stopping to think about it. We use it to cover all sorts of difficult situations. It comes on slowly or may slam us without warning. Either way, it seems difficult to avoid. It doesn't have to be that way.

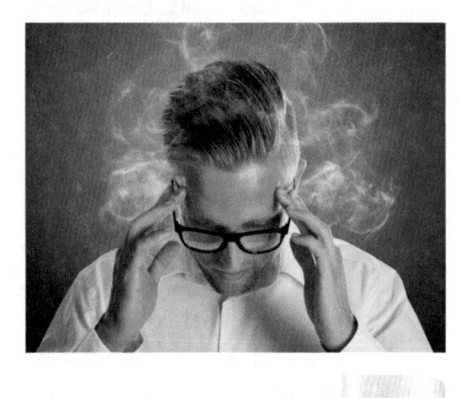

> *Do not be anxious about anything, but in everything by prayer and supplication with thanksgiving let your requests be made known to God. And the peace of God, which surpasses all understanding, will guard your hearts and your minds in Christ Jesus.*
>
> **Philippians 4:6-7**

Intuitively, we are right. Stress that we experience is a **direct response** to what we perceive as tense, dangerous, or unknown situations. However, even though we perceive stress as something that happens in our heads, the truth is that stress is primarily a physical reaction.

 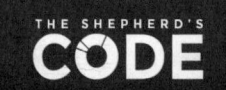

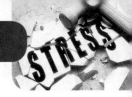

We can divide stress into **psychological and biological (or physical, physiological) components**. Biological stress is what happens in our bodies when we are faced with a sudden and dangerous situation or an injury – adrenaline and other hormones kick in, our heart rate goes up, we spring into action and tend to think less.

Psychological stress is that continuous feeling of strain and pressure that we feel, and what we usually refer to in our everyday talk. These two components are not mutually exclusive, but a part of a larger system. For the sake of simplicity, let's refer to the whole system as simply stress from this point onward. We won't make a terrible mistake, as these components are intertwined and negatively influence our lives in an equal measure.

So, how exactly does stress impact our health?

Let's start with our minds:

As of 2016, there were over **40 million adults in the US affected by anxiety**, according to the National Institute of Mental Health, as well as millions more who have been afflicted with depression-related disorders. Almost one in five Americans has some form of mental illness. While it is certain that genetics and environment play a role, most of these cases of anxiety, depression, and other disorders have stress as one of the main causes.

> Even scarier, stress could be a potential factor in serious diseases where there is a physical degradation of the brain. One study on Alzheimer's disease suggests exactly this.

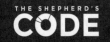

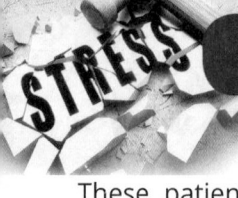

These patients were mostly aged sixty to eighty and they led significantly more stressful lives than their healthy counterparts in control the group. According to the lead researcher and author, Dr. Edgardo Reich, this study has potentially worrying consequences:

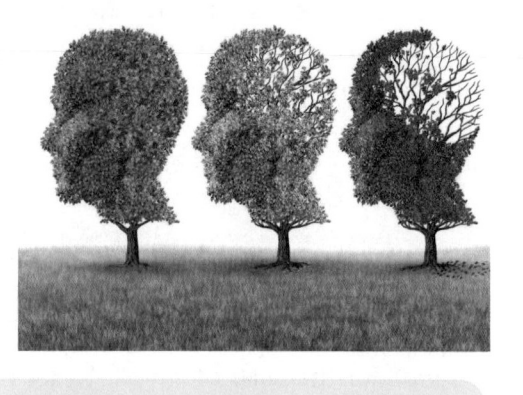

"**Stress,** according to our findings, is probably **a trigger for initial symptoms of dementia**. Though I rule out stress as monocausal in dementia, research is solidifying the evidence that stress can trigger a degenerative process in the brain and precipitate dysfunction in the neuroendocrine and immune system. It is an observational finding and does not imply direct causality. Further studies are needed to examine these mechanisms in detail."

OUR PHYSICAL HEALTH

No matter how terrible and scary these statistics and implications are, it is only the tip of the iceberg. Stress also puts a huge strain on our bodies. It is one of the factors that lead to obesity and buildup of visceral fat, also known as belly fat. **Visceral fat** is a type of fat that is stored in the abdominal or stomach area, and it fills the gaps between our organs and pads them in layers of this semi-liquid kind of unhealthy fat. This seems an awful way to live and it is, until we

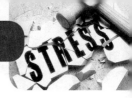

can find rest knowing we have tools to combat these issues AND the promise of what is to come. Until then, we are wise to recognize the warning signs and take steps to reverse the symptoms of our lifestyles.

> *And after you have suffered a little while, the God of all grace, who has called you to his eternal glory in Christ, will himself restore, confirm, strengthen, and establish you.*
>
> **1 Peter 5:10**

Visceral fat is linked to type 2 diabetes, insulin resistance, various inflammatory diseases, and other serious health issues.

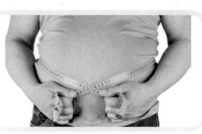

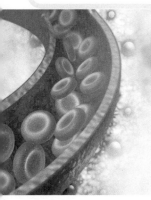

This type of fat is extremely damaging to our health as it can **enter our bloodstream and clog our arteries,** enter our organs and reduce their functioning...

While this fat is more common in men due to the differences in male and female sex hormones, women are far from safe. Even if they are fairly slim or have most of their

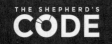

fat stored in the form of cellulite under their skin, this epidermal fat also tends to migrate upward and turn into visceral fat when menopause kicks in.

Furthermore, a study done at Yale University suggests that stress is directly connected to creation of belly fat in otherwise slim middle-aged women. One of the observations made by the lead researcher, Elissa S. Epel, Ph.D., explained the reason these women experienced this problem:

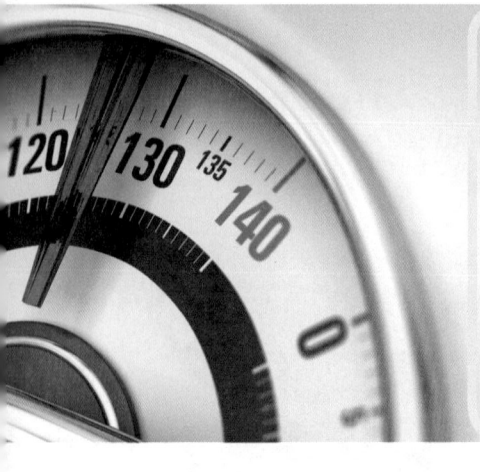

"[However,] excess weight on men is almost always stored at the abdomen. On the contrary, in premenopausal women, excess weight is more often stored at the hips. Therefore, for women, it is possible that stress may influence body shape more than for men, leading to abdominal fat instead of lower body fat accumulation."

Obesity and fat are not the only health concerns that can be influenced by stress. Actually, it might be the least of our concerns, in this case.

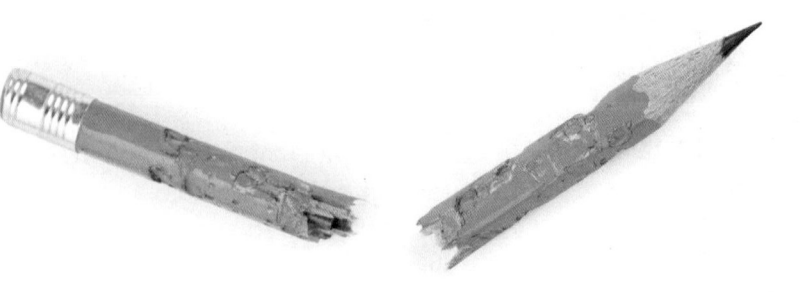

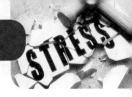

Stress has been linked to such an astounding number of issues that affect almost every system in the human body that it would simply sound unbelievable if there weren't studies upon studies done on the subject.

**Just to illustrate,
stress has been linked to:**

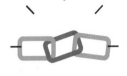

1 **Gastrointestinal issues**, like irritable bowel syndrome (IBS), diarrhea or constipation, heartburn (acid reflux), nausea, and so on.

2 **Cardiovascular (heart) and respiratory problems**, such as inflammation of arteries (which are believed to be a potential cause of a heart attack), hyperventilation (fast, panicked, breathing) and panic attacks.

3 Improper functioning of our **reproductive system**, both female and male. Stress can cause impotence and lower sperm count in men, and irregular, absent, and more painful menstrual cycles in women.

4 **Migraines, fatigue, frequent urination, and allergies** are also linked to stress in some cases, and this list goes on and on.

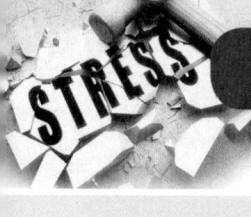
To understand how this all can happen, and how stress can affect our minds and bodies so much, let's take a look at one of the culprits, cortisol.

WHAT IS CORTISOL?

Or do you not know that your body is a temple of the Holy Spirit within you, whom you have from God? You are not your own,

1 Corinthians 6:19

When we remember that our bodies are way more than the vehicle for getting through life, we suddenly have renewed desire to care for it well. The Holy Spirit is just that--holy, set apart, and worthy of only the best. As stewards of a flesh and bone body, it becomes our responsibility to identify the junk and keep it away from our body temple!

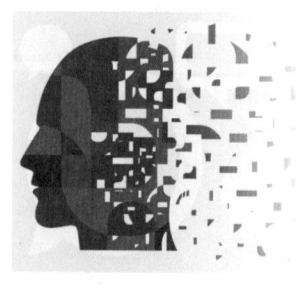

Cortisol is a hormone like adrenalin that is released when we feel threatened. It is your body's reply to that fight or flight instinct. Its primary purpose is to ramp up production of glucose so that our muscles can have enough energy to deal with the dangerous situation. In addition, it reduces inflammation.

 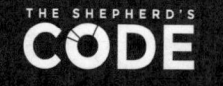

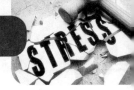

Cortisol is created by **breaking down cholesterol,** so you might think that all of this sounds pretty good. But the thing is, cortisol is extremely damaging if its levels do not decrease over time, most commonly due to prolonged stress.

Cortisol's primary concern is **to get enough sugar in our blood at all costs.** This means that it will break down protein – it will start to burn your muscles for fuel. It also tends to do the same with bones over time, leading to osteoporosis and thinning of your bones.

It also breaks down fat. Which might sound good, but it **actually breaks down less dangerous fat** that is stored under our skin and converts it into dangerous visceral fat. Oh, and it also counteracts insulin.

Since it negates the effects of insulin, it can also lead to insulin resistance, which is bad news for everybody, particularly if you're diabetic. **It suppresses the immune system** in a number of ways making us sicker overall and it also greatly increases wound healing and recovery time.

And, of course, it also **impairs your brain function.** Prolonged exposure to cortisol has been shown to damage cells in certain areas of our brains, leading to impaired learning capabilities and difficulties in remembering things.

When we are suffering from chronic stress and anxiety, **our bodies become less sensitive to cortisol.** Since one of the purposes of cortisol is to reduce inflammation, we actually become more vulnerable to it, even with the heightened level of cortisol in our blood. Inflammation is a bad thing, and it can lead to heart diseases, cancer, Alzheimer's, and other terrible and lethal illnesses.

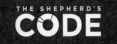

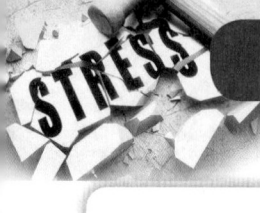

The list goes on and on. It's obvious that cortisol is bad news. As if all of this wasn't enough, remember how cortisol increases sugar levels in your blood?

This is exactly what we're trying to avoid when you begin your new lifestyle by eating "healing fats" and avoiding unhealthy fats.

The Shepherd's Code is based on the idea that we force our bodies to use ketone bodies as our fuel source instead of glucose. In order to do that, we need to have very limited amounts of carbohydrates.

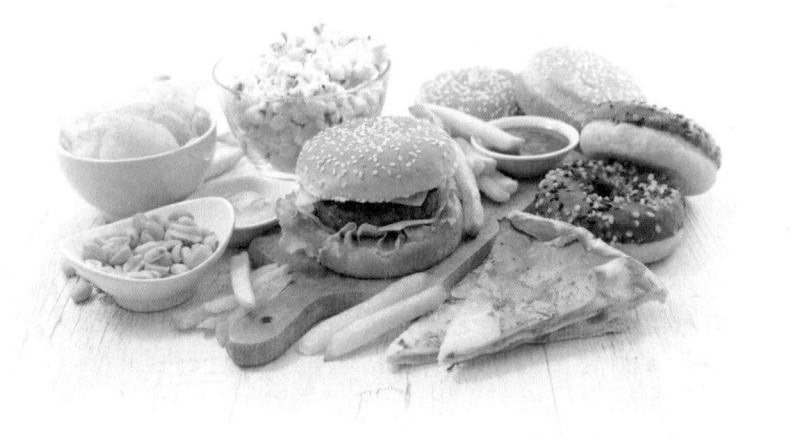

So, the problem is that cortisol will break down muscle and fat to create glucose, thus preventing your body to enter ketosis and start burning fat as a fuel source.

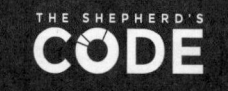

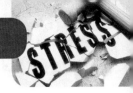

 Luckily, cortisol is not all-powerful. Even though it greatly impairs the efficiency of the low-carb diet, ketone bodies have such a positive impact on your energy levels and your physical and mental health that they greatly reduce stress (both biological and psychological), and we experience lowered cortisol levels, which in turns increases your diet's efficiency, and thus the positive loop is formed.

A diet heavy in "healing fats" has antioxidant properties, not unlike those that are attributed to that famous "one glass of wine per day". This is important because oxidants are very **damaging to our cells**, and are one of the main reasons why we age. Even though we need oxygen to live, it is an unfortunate irony that it also slowly kills us over time due to these "free radicals".

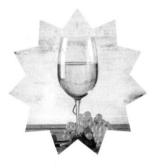

HOW TO APPROACH STRESS

? **Why does stress, a supposedly vital reaction to our survival, have negative effect on us?**

It's rather simple:

We were never designed to experience stress for prolonged periods of time. In the ancient times, when humans first walked the Earth, stress was a part of our fight or flight response, it reduced inflammation, and made us able to live to another day.

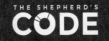

But it would happen only occasionally, when something endangered our survival.

Today, we are actually commanded not to have anxiety about anything. That sounds impossible, but when we learn to reduce or eliminate stress by handing it over to the One for whom all things are possible, **it begins to make sense.** There is transformative, restorative power in prayer. I urge you to lean into your faith while you take this journey into learning more about yourself and how you've been fearfully and wonderfully made.

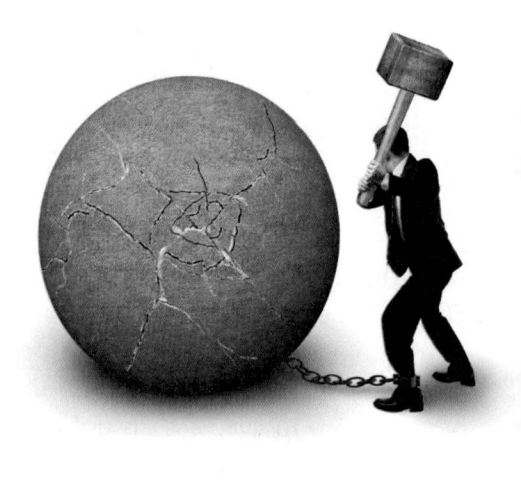

Do not be anxious about anything, but in everything by prayer and supplication with thanksgiving let your requests be made known to God.

Philippians 4:6

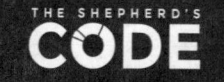

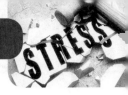

In the modern day society, stress is unavoidable. We meet such a diverse group of people on a daily basis, all with their own values and opinions. We face deadlines and pressure to excel at our jobs, lest we be fired.

In other words, we go through all the typical human experiences like getting hurt, losing loved ones, providing for our families, and so on. Even though these situations are in reality much less dangerous than being chased by a saber tooth tiger, our subconscious identifies them as threats and acts accordingly. We feel the pressure all the time.

 Now more than ever, a modern human feels troubled.

The American Psychological Association (APA) has found that over 50% of Americans were stressed about recent presidential elections. Furthermore, with the rise of violence and the threat of terrorism, **we feel less safe than ever**. Even without eminent danger our fears of negative potential cause turmoil inside of us. Believe it or not, that's not all bad.

Anxiety in a man's heart weighs him down, but a good word makes him glad.

Proverbs 12:25

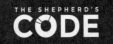

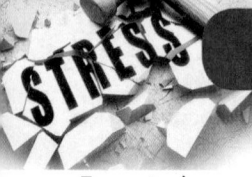
Even today, small amounts of stress can have positive effects, which is **good news**, since stress is unavoidable. We must not let stress take over our lives, though.

Before we delve into different ways to reduce stress, it is important that we understand a few things:

 Stress is normal.

It is literally impossible not to feel stress. In small doses, it can have a positive effect on our health and performance (better known as eustress). Maybe you've experienced the situation where you procrastinate until the last minute. Then, suddenly, you finish a project or an assignment in a fraction of the time you thought you would need, under seemingly divine inspiration? That feeling of stress made sure you finished it.

 **Stress is relative.**

Objective danger is not a problem when we talk about our stress; our perception of it is the real problem. One of the biggest issues with stress is how relative it is. We feel like we shouldn't be stressed about something because others aren't (or even worse, they might be, but we think they are not). This frame of mind makes us feel like we are weak, or unworthy, and further adds to the stress.

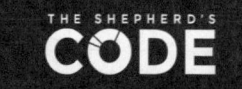

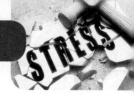

We need to accept these two statements and what they mean for us. It's ok to feel stress. There is nothing wrong with you if you do… but you do have a choice about how much stress you feel and how you manage it. I'll show you ten tips for how to do it in a few seconds.

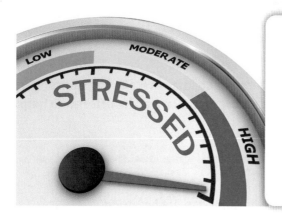

It is also ok if a seemingly insignificant situation is putting you under a lot of stress.

That situation is important to you, and we all react to stress differently. There is no absolute value for feeling stressed or things that should or should not make you feel that way.

Now, we must not let stress overwhelm us and take over. If we are under continuous tension, bad things start to happen to our bodies and minds; we start to feel tired, depressed, anxious, and in general feel bad about ourselves.

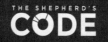

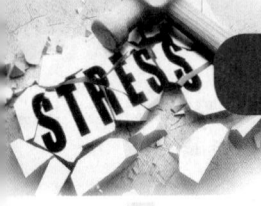
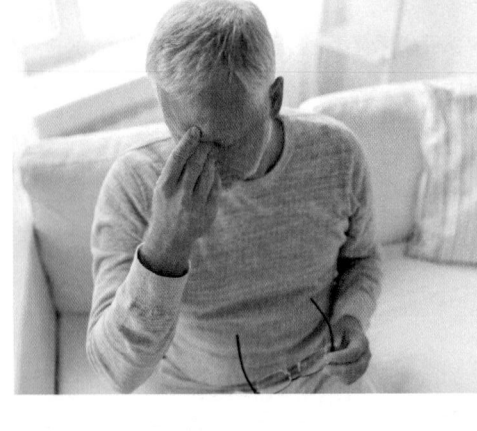

We stress about being stressed.

We push away others or lash out at them. These feelings feed on each other, and we enter a negative cycle of behaviors.

We are not without hope. There are solid answers to the question of how to deal with stress. **Jesus said it plainly when he offered to help:**

Come to me, all who labor and are heavy laden, and I will give you rest. Take my yoke upon you, and learn from me, for I am gentle and lowly in heart, and you will find rest for your souls. For my yoke is easy, and my burden is light.

Matthew 11:28-30

 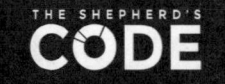

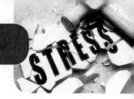

10 TIPS TO REDUCE STRESS AND ANXIETY

The first step in helping relieve the anxiety and depression naturally leads from this:

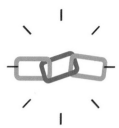

1. HAVE THE RIGHT MINDSET

It's extremely important to understand how you feel and accept it when you are anxious, depressed, sad, worried, and so on. It takes an honest and humble heart to be able to recognize emotions and passions for what they are. Some of these feelings are the open door for Satan to get a foothold in your life. Keep close guard over your self!

> *Be sober-minded; be watchful. Your adversary the devil prowls around like a roaring lion, seeking someone to devour.*
>
> **1 Peter 5:8**

Even with all that doom and gloom, it can often be surprisingly easy to break this negative loop.

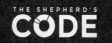

Now that we've discussed how to enter a bit better and more open mindset, we can take a look at some of the ways we can relax, wind down, and alleviate our concerns.

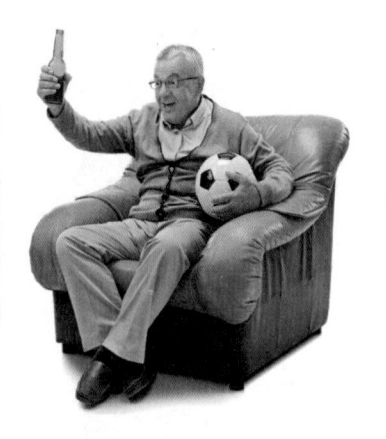

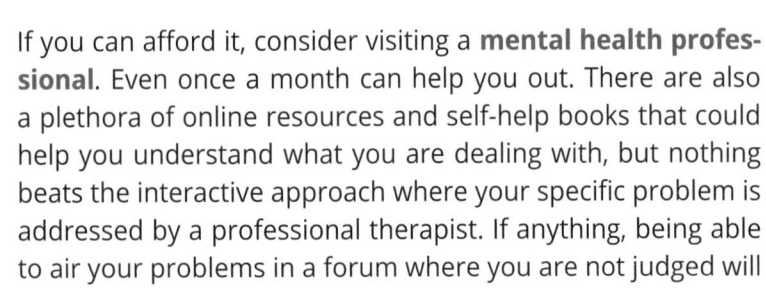

*Remember, **understanding what is going on with you is very important.** You can't relax while watching a movie or playing with your children if you've got that nagging feeling at the back of your mind that something is wrong.*

2. HAVE SOMEONE TO TALK WITH

If you can afford it, consider visiting a **mental health professional**. Even once a month can help you out. There are also a plethora of online resources and self-help books that could help you understand what you are dealing with, but nothing beats the interactive approach where your specific problem is addressed by a professional therapist. If anything, being able to air your problems in a forum where you are not judged will always relieve some stress.

Alternatively, have a few friends over or join a small group Bible study through your church or community. It is important to verbalize your concerns and let them out in the open. When you do that, when you acknowledge those fears, and their significance and power over you become greatly diminished.

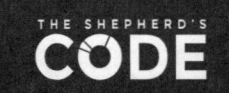

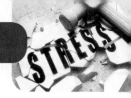

> *Bear one another's burdens, and so fulfill the law of Christ.*
>
> **Galatians 6:2**

In addition, **hanging out** with other people is truly important to our wellbeing. Loneliness is an incredibly damaging feeling, and some studies show that it is more of a health risk than obesity.

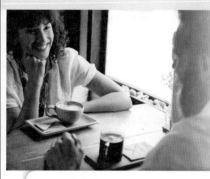

Today, even if you do not have friends, it is easier than ever to find **like-minded people**. You can simply search online for a group that is interested in something you are.

Forums, Facebook groups like *The Shepherd's Code*, **www.shepcodefamily.com**, and other websites are all viable options, and you can either meet new people that way or at least find information where various events are happening in your neighborhood.

Consider **getting a pet**. Our furry friends, like cats and dogs, have been scientifically proven to reduce stress. Dogs are also valuable because they require you to be more physically active and go outside every day, both of which can help in alleviating depression and other mental issues.

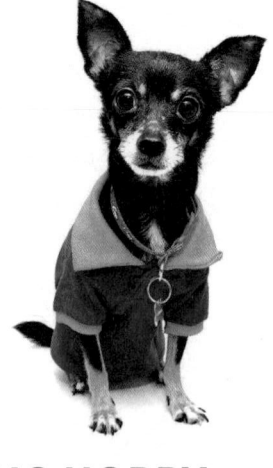

3. CONSIDER A RELAXING HOBBY

Also that everyone should eat and drink and take pleasure in all his toil — this is God's gift to man.

Ecclesiastes 3:13

There is so much to see, do, and enjoy in God's creation. Whether mountains, water, sun, or sand, there are many places where you can find the peace that comes from being surrounded by nature and experiencing what was made not by the hands of man.

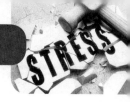

Finding comfort in something that you love is the oldest trick in the book. Hobbies that require concentration and slow repetitive movements like **whittling, knitting, sewing, golf or tennis** can be an amazing way to calm yourself down. In fact, any kind of creative outlet, like painting, writing, and playing music can be a great way to relieve some stress and anxiety.

Organizing things is also relaxing to some, so any type of collecting hobby can be an interesting option.

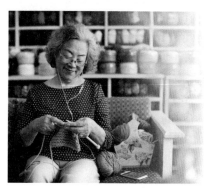

Of course, hobbies like fishing, bird watching, gardening, and landscape photography that are not physically demanding but force you to spend time outside are beneficial.

The main takeaway here is to do whatever you like and find relaxing; there are no rules to abide by here.

4. FIND A SAFE SPACE

As we said, most stress comes from feeling a sense of danger, whether real or not. We feel unsafe, and we have a need to protect ourselves. This is a perfectly normal and sane response when you think about it. Even if we can't identify what makes us feel so unsafe, we can still soothe our subconscious a little bit.

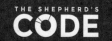

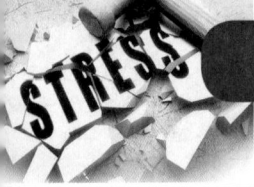
Find, or create, a place where **you feel safe** and peaceful. It can be anywhere and anything as long as it makes you feel safe.

Try to create a daily routine where you commit at least 10-15 minutes to staying in your safe and peaceful place and pay attention to how it makes you feel. Chances are, this will make you feel rejuvenated, and you will feel calmer.

For some this "place" won't be so much a destination as a state of mind. With your eyes closed and ears covered, you may find simply cutting out the "noise" is something that takes practice but helps you release the earthly bindings **that seem to strangle and restrict our lives**.

He who dwells in the shelter of the Most High will abide in the shadow of the Almighty. I will say to the Lord, "My refuge and my fortress, my God, in whom I trust." For he will deliver you from the snare of the fowler and from the deadly pestilence. He will cover you with his pinions, and under his wings you will find refuge; his faithfulness is a shield and buckler. You will not fear the terror of the night, nor the arrow that flies by day, ...

Psalm 91:1-16

 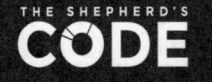

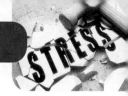

5. MEDITATE

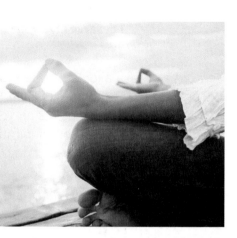

In a similar manner to a safe space, meditation can help you create an inner safe space. Clearing your mind for even ten minutes a day can have an amazing effect on your wellbeing. There are a huge number of different types of meditation, but don't be intimidated, just try to find the one that you are most comfortable with.

Having the words to reflect on and becoming adept at meditation means you will be able to soothe yourself more easily no matter where you are or what is going on.

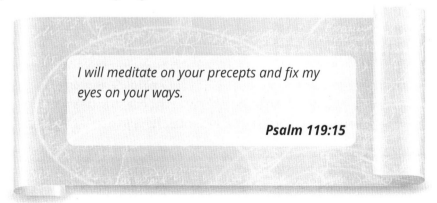

I will meditate on your precepts and fix my eyes on your ways.

Psalm 119:15

In addition, you can try various self-approval methods like repeating a certain positive, empowering message to yourself.

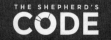

> *Depending on your situation and source of stress and anxiety, you can go with statements like **"I am safe"**, **"I am worthy"**, **"I deserve my success"**, **"Others like me"**, and so on...*

You can also take a look at various alternative practices like the Emotional Freedom Technique (EFT). In EFT you relieve stress by tapping on various acupressure points on your body while trying to empower yourself through verbal communication. Even if you're skeptical about this sort of thing, it's worth checking out as a lot of people find that this technique helps them a lot.

6. EXERCISE

Even ancient Romans believed in the power of exercise. "Mens sana in corpore sano " is a Latin proverb that means **"healthy mind in a healthy body"**. And Romans were definitely on to something, as even light daily physical activity reduces stress, increases endorphins, and helps us in general.

A simple brisk walk every day can lift your spirits. Swimming is a great way to stay active and lose some weight, and it doesn't stress your joints, so it's a great activity if you're overweight or have joint pain or injuries.

If you feel **more ambitious**, you can start going to yoga classes or have light gym sessions. If you're feeling insecure about your body or your weight, don't worry. No one will laugh at you for trying to get better. In fact, people always appreciate and support such a desire. After all, they all come to such places with the same goal as you:
To get healthier and in better shape.

 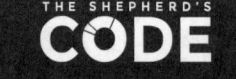

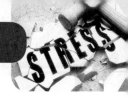

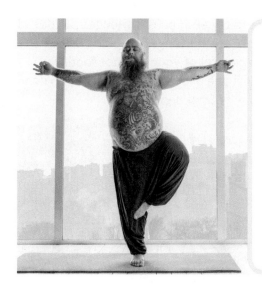

Even so, I suggest that you find a smaller studio or a gym, as trainers will be able to pay more attention to you (especially if you can't or don't want to pay for personal training), and there is a certain sense of camaraderie in such small places that can make you feel more comfortable overall.

7. EAT A HEALTHY DIET

The miracle of a healthy diet should not be foreign to you; after all, you decided to change your life by joining over 100,000 others on their journey to better health. Eating well and not overeating puts less stress on our bodies, gives us more energy, and boosts our immune system. Not only does this reduce physical stress, it also makes us feel better ourselves.

Fortunately, a diet primarily focused on eating "healing fats" and low in carbohydrates **helps reduce stress on your biological system and your brain.**

With a high carbohydrate diet, your body and mind are constantly burning sugar and looking for more to keep the "high." When your body

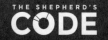

burns fat, you have sustained energy and focus for longer periods of time, and you stay satiated. **You are no longer thinking about the next snack or meal. You are in control of your life, not food!**

And, feeling good about yourself is one of the best things you can do to calm down anxiety and get yourself out of depression.

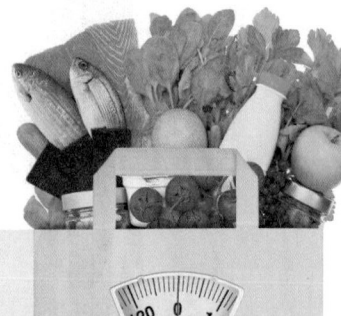

You can't always cure severe clinical depression, anxiety or any other sort of pathological state simply by eating well.

However, even in these cases, a proper diet will surely help a lot in reducing the severity and frequency of symptoms.

Don't forget to **hydrate.** Drink around two liters of water per day, if possible. Even though it may sound like a lot, you don't even feel it if you drink it throughout the whole day. The best way is to have a pitcher or a bottle that you sip from every now and then. That way, you won't feel bloated, and water retention is much better; more of it hydrates your cells instead of just passing quickly through your body.

8. HOT BATHS AND HOT BEVERAGES

Pamper yourself. Find some time every now and then to enjoy. Make yourself a hot bath, or curl up with some nice green or chamomile tea, listen to some relaxing music, watch a nice movie or a show, read a book, or do whatever

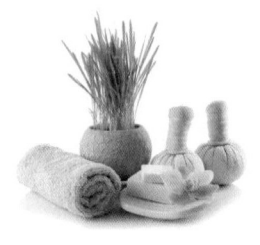

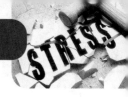

you find relaxing. Most importantly, don't feel guilty about having some time for yourself. I find that the serenity of a bath or luxurious massage is an opportunity for "deep detoxification". These are times when I can better recognize, ask forgiveness for, and let go of feelings that hurt, intentions that are misguided, and then I can begin to pour love back out instead of negativity.

> *If we confess our sins, he is faithful and just to forgive us our sins and to cleanse us from all unrighteousness.*
>
> **1 John 1:9**

If you can afford it, go to a spa or have a massage. Sometimes, it is easiest to get out of the house for a while if you're having energetic kids or roommates around.

9. DANCE AND LISTEN TO MUSIC

 Last but not least, have fun! Dance, even if you're alone.

In fact, especially if you're alone. **Let go, crank your favorite tunes and go to town!** There's no shame in it and from it come many blessings!

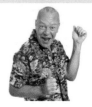

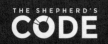

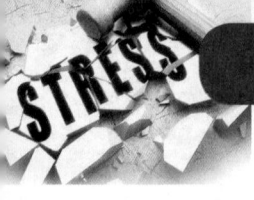

> *Then shall the young women rejoice in the dance, and the young men and the old shall be merry. I will turn their mourning into joy; I will comfort them, and give them gladness for sorrow.*
>
> **Jeremiah 31:13**

Dancing is great for you because it is both a physical activity and a social behavior. Slow dancing with your partner releases a hormone called oxytocin, commonly known as the love, or cuddle, hormone.

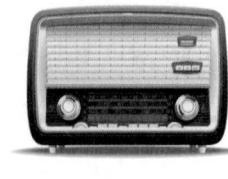

Dancing in general is a very liberating experience and a great way to release some of that pent-up stress and anxiety.

10. SLEEP WELL

After all the activities mentioned in this list, it is only natural that you would need some rest. Sleep is an incredibly important part of our health, and it is obvious that we need rest in order to have energy. There is no up without down and no good work without rest. Savor your time to recharge. It too is a gift.

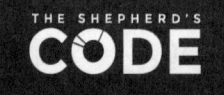

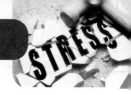

> *For everything there is a season, and a time for every matter under heaven: a time to be born, and a time to die; a time to plant, and a time to pluck up what is planted; a time to kill, and a time to heal; a time to break down, and a time to build up; a time to weep, and a time to laugh; a time to mourn, and a time to dance; a time to cast away stones, and a time to gather stones together; a time to embrace, and a time to refrain from embracing; ...*
>
> **Ecclesiastes 3:1-22**

Ideally, you would get between six and eight hours of sleep per day, and it would be at the same time. It is key to have a fixed sleeping schedule, as it allows your circadian rhythm to operate properly.

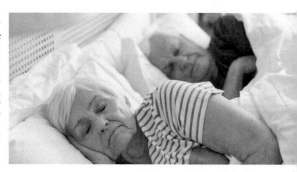

In simplest terms, circadian rhythm represents various phases our bodies go through throughout the day. For example, before we go to sleep, our body starts to slow our metabolism down, various physical processes change their mode of operation, and we get into "repair and

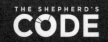

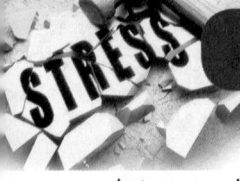
maintenance" mode. When we are to wake up naturally, our inner clock sets off an alarm, and we get flooded with various hormones that increase our activity and alertness.

> If you've ever wondered why you are so drowsy when someone (or an alarm) wakes you mid-slumber, **it is for that exact reason–your body didn't have time to prepare for waking up.**

This is, of course, greatly simplified, and there are many more things that happen throughout the day, but you get the idea.

In order **to get good sleep**, it would be best if your room is moderately cold, dark, and quiet. White noise, like the hum of the fan or air-conditioning is not a problem as it is constant. In addition, avoid watching TV, using computers, smartphones and similar devices several hours before going to bed. Screens from our electronics emit a lot of blue light which signals our body that it is still day.

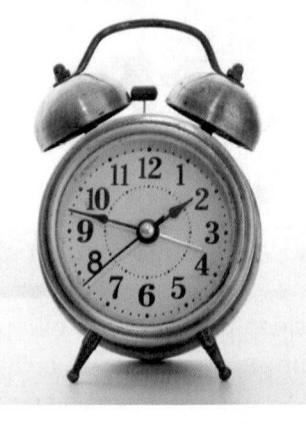

If you always feel exhausted after sleep, consult a medical professional. You might have sleep apnea, restless leg syndrome, or some other sort of sleep disorder.

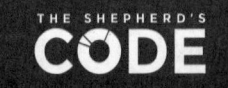

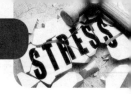

CONCLUSION

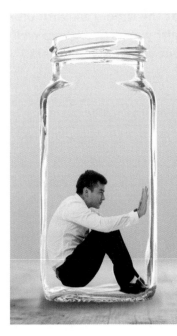

Stress is literally a killer. The worst part of it is not a vast number of different consequences that have different effects on our lives; the worst part is that we do it to ourselves. In order to live long and healthy lives, we need to take a deep breath, say that it's ok to make mistakes, and understand that we are far from perfect.

You are not perfect, and neither is anyone else on this planet. We are defined by relationships, and it is natural that the opinions of others matter to us. But there is nothing scary about that. Even when we are faced with difficult decisions and choices, we have to trust that we will do our best.

I'm not saying that it's easy, that everything is rainbows and butterflies, no. Life can be hard and devastating. At times, we have full right to be stressed, overwhelmed, miserable, and anxious.

But we have to accept this, and **deal with it in our own imperfect ways**.

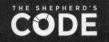

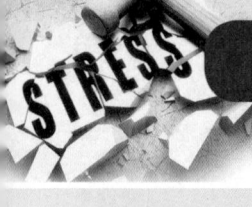
We need to love and accept ourselves first, and to do that, we need to work on our quality of life, one step at the time. Talk with others, enjoy things that you enjoy, eat healthy, exercise, sleep well, and try to learn as much as possible about yourself and others.

So, take a deep breath, say that everything will be ok, and **start believing it.**

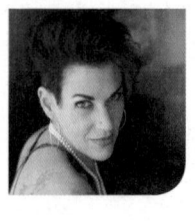

All things are possible!

Kristina Wilds

CELEBRITY ANTI-AGING & WEIGHT LOSS SECRET

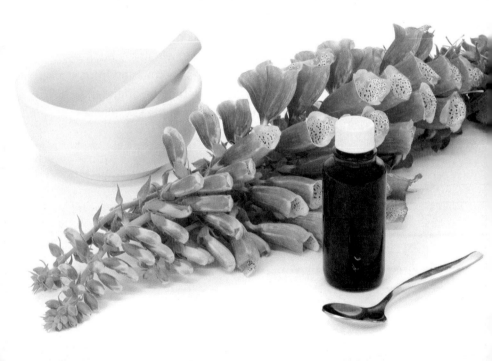

THE SHEPHERD'S
CODE

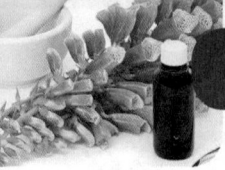

The contents of this document are based upon my opinions of *The Shepherd's Code* unless otherwise noted. This work is intended to share knowledge and information learned through research, experience, and discussions with others. The opinions of others, such as in the comments and the forum, are their own and are not endorsed by *The Shepherd's Code*. The information contained herein is not intended to diagnose, treat, cure or prevent any condition or disease, but rather to provide general information that is intended to be used for educational purposes only. Please consult with your physician or healthcare practitioner if you have any concerns. By using, viewing and interacting with *The Shepherd's Code* or **shepherdscode.com** website, you agree to all terms of engagement, thus assuming complete responsibility for your own actions. The authors and publishers will not claim accountability, nor shall they be held liable for any loss or injury sustained by you. Use, view and interact with these resources at your own risk. All products and information given to you by *The Shepherd's Code* and its related companies are strictly for informational purposes only. While every attempt has been made to verify the accuracy of information provided on our website and within our publications, neither the authors nor the publishers are responsible for assuming liability for possible inaccuracies. The authors and publishers disclaim any responsibility for the inaccuracy of the content, including but not limited to errors or omissions. Loss of property, injury to self or others, and even death could occur as a direct or indirect consequence of the use and application of any content found herein. Please act responsibly. The information provided may need to be downloaded and/or viewed using third party software, such as Acrobat. It's the user's responsibility to install the software necessary to view such information. Any downloads, whether purchased or given for free from our website, related websites or hosting systems are performed at the user's own risk. Although we take great preventative measures, we cannot warranty that our websites are free of corrupting computer codes, viruses or worms. If you are a minor, you can use this service only with permission and guidance from your parents or guardians.

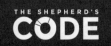

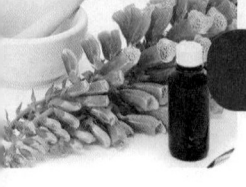

I appeal to you therefore, brothers, by the mercies of God, to present your bodies as a living sacrifice, holy and acceptable to God, which is your spiritual worship. Do not be conformed to this world,but be transformed by the renewal of your mind, that by testing you may discern what is the will of God, what is good and acceptable and perfect.

Romans 12:1-2

For the many of us who gaze wide-eyed at the celebrities on the silver screen or in the pages of a magazine, it's easy to assume that achieving beauty like theirs must be as costly as their designer clothes. When specialized skin treatments and personalized formulas are only obtained by way of costly appointments and prescriptions, achieving that youthful glow becomes an expensive and exhausting effort.

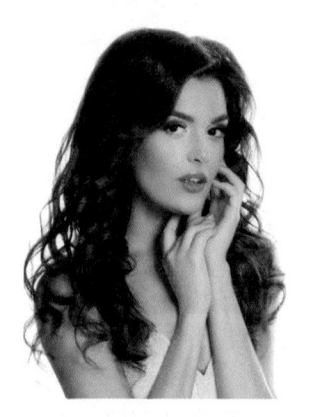

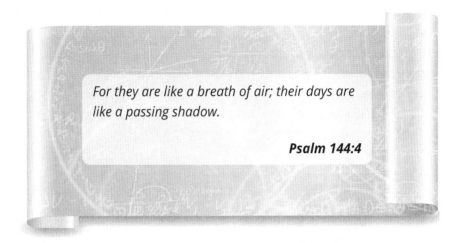

For they are like a breath of air; their days are like a passing shadow.

Psalm 144:4

But, If only we had celebrity status and the bankroll to show for it. Then we too would have access to the experts and their miracle complexion cures. Right? Wrong!

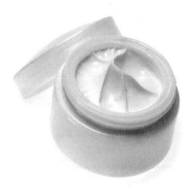

The world of skincare marketing has grown wise to the manipulation game and they play it well. With words and images they twist reality to convince us that their product alone is the gateway to the smooth, radiant, and healthy skin we long for.

Celebrities who are paid for their endorsement of skincare products go along with the story because it's written into their contracts. Of course they're going to smile and recite their lines--it's what they do!

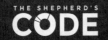

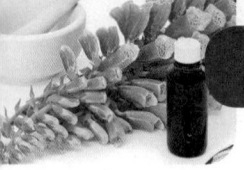

The skincare industry pulls in close to a billion dollars every year. With that kind of reinforcement, it's not solutions to skin problems that drives these companies' efforts. Rather, it is whatever will keep that money rolling in. They'd be out of business pretty quickly if everyone's skin became healed. So, therefore, false claims and doctored images hide the destructive truth behind all the lotions and potions they push so hard to get into our hands.

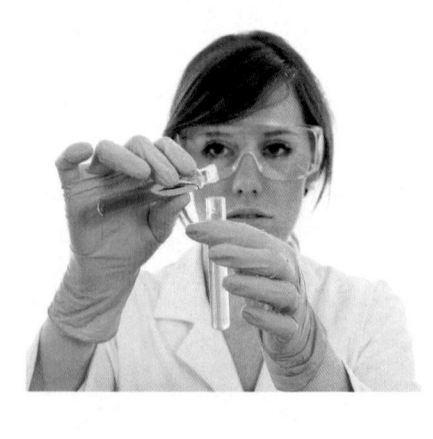

With ever increasing "research" on anti-aging, isn't it amazing that our personal stockpiles of skincare products STILL aren't getting the job done? That's because so many of us are out there chasing an illusion, an illusion that costs a fortune!

The reality that you are about to discover in this book is transformative. You will learn how going back to basics, and understanding your skin, debunks all the myths you've been tricked into believing.

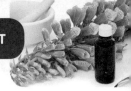

YOUR SKIN, YOUR SELF

Your skin is a bodily organ with many important functions. Luckily, our skin needs only a few basic requirements to help it function well. For example, the skin responds better to less manipulation rather than more. Skin is appropriately very sensitive and may become irritated or damaged by harsh ingredients, environment, stress, etc.. Following a daily regimen like that exposes you to the aging you don't want!

Are you ready for the transformation that awaits you? Keep reading to experience the inspiration for each step toward restoring youthful skin. We'll unravel the celebrity secret that makes everyone look so fresh and young. These techniques are not reserved for the rich and famous. This is something we can all do to feel new.

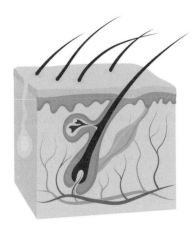

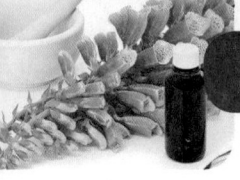

BACK TO BASICS

> Different skin requires a different approach.

Change creates change.
First, we need to change
how we view the care of
our skin.

Celebrities get paid to look good
and are encouraged to maintain their
healthy glow and smooth features. Many even
claim to use the products they endorse, but if that were the case,
wouldn't we all look like a million bucks? After all, plenty of us shell out
for those name brand products the celebrity names are attached to.

It's easy to fall into the traps set by big names, bright lights, and what
looks to be a glamourous lifestyle. But while smoke and mirrors paint
a picture we think is beautiful, it's that deception that can serve as our
undoing. The Lord has given you exactly what he has intended you to
work with, to become refined by, and to enjoy to it's fullest. Your own
home, your own face, body, and circle of influence is where you can
shine most brightly and find true blessings. We can choose to find con-
tentment and health with even the simplest of means.

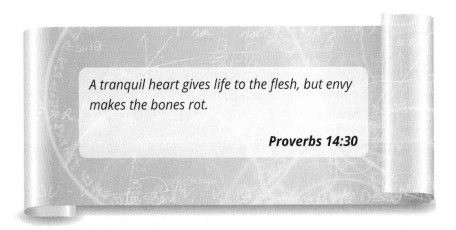

A tranquil heart gives life to the flesh, but envy makes the bones rot.

Proverbs 14:30

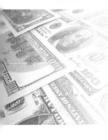

If everyone saw how just pennies a day could afford the skin care that truly reveals healthy, glowing skin, those huge companies would fall overnight! So, what does it take? What is the routine that can set us free from harsh chemicals and blind faith in false claims?

It has taken the collaborative efforts of some of Hollywood's greatest minds to sift through the rubbish to discover what actually works. Trade secrets from dermatologists, stylists, and health care professionals have been put together to create the ultimate routine. At last, this perfect method is available to the masses. Now, you can transform the skin you're in--to it's beautiful best, as it was meant to be.

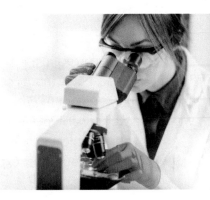

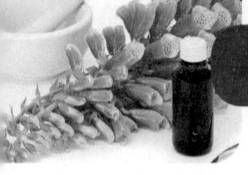
Faces showing years of neglect or abuse will heal with the single routine that works for all skin types. Acne scars, wrinkles, sagging, discoloration, dryness, and blemishes will all find this simple detoxifying process the means to amazing transformation. What's best of all, is that secret is for everyone! Both affordable and safe, these steps will give generations new life!

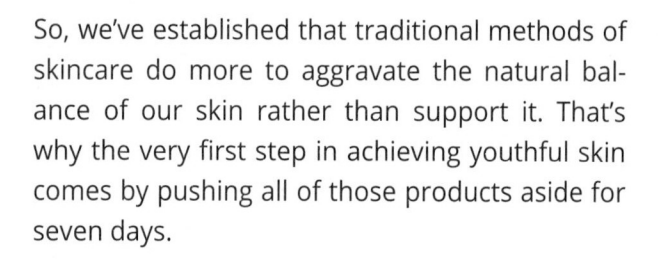

Allowing this healing to begin is a breeze. Let us guide you through each chapter as we lay out the support and instructions you need to help it happen.

THE ONE WEEK SKIN DETOX

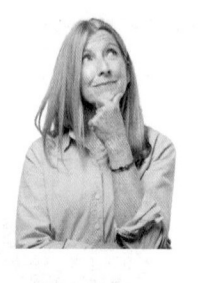

So, we've established that traditional methods of skincare do more to aggravate the natural balance of our skin rather than support it. That's why the very first step in achieving youthful skin comes by pushing all of those products aside for seven days.

You may be correct in thinking that you know your own skin better than anyone else, but without chemical interference, you may find your skin tells an entirely different story. Your commitment to transformation will be well rewarded. Feed your excitement and curiosity and see just what your complexion reveals in just one week. You very well may find that giving up your most expensive treatments improves the health of your skin in days!

Oh, I know how hard it is to discredit even the "truths" about skincare and wellness that we've come to hold so dear. After all, we structure our lives around certain beliefs about food, health, and what we deem to be morally right and wrong about certain methods of beautification and preservation. But there is no growth without change, and you'll never know unless you try.

> *Be not wise in your own eyes; fear the Lord, and turn away from evil. It will be healing to your flesh and refreshment to your bones.*
>
> **Proverbs 3:7-8**

We are taught that there is healing and refreshment when wisdom comes not from external influence, but from the Lord. His ways are pure and he's made you in such a way that nothing more was needed to "improve" his design of YOU. Let's be rid of the junk and find what beauty lies beneath.

To detox your skin properly you must promise yourself freedom from ANY and EVERY facial product. That includes soap, moisturizer, toner, and any other product other than pure water. Anything else has the potential to affect your skin's reaction to both internal and external influences.

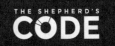

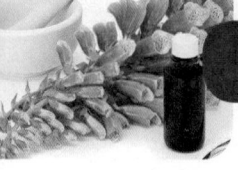

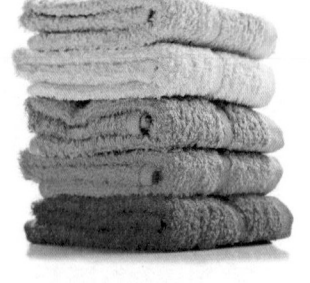

Now you're wondering how to keep your face clean without cleansers? The most natural formula out there is really quite simple! Twice a day you will use plain luke-warm water on a clean cloth to gently dab and freshen your face. Always use clean hands that have been rinsed of any soap or lotions. Purity is key here, so try your best to keep your hands off of your face throughout the day unless it is absolutely necessary.

Defense is your plan for seven days of truly clean skin. Journaling your observations may help you reveal more than just surface changes. Don't be dismayed if the initial changes don't seem positive. The purging process takes time to run its course. An effective detox may seem to actually throw things off before they become balanced. Yet, within a weeks time, your skin will have leached out remaining toxins and be ready for a fresh start.

H₂O

Drawing out and removing the triggers that make our skin act up is essential, but it's not the only key to achieving that anti-aging power celebrities wear so well. After a complexion chemical detox, all that's been stripped away needs replacement by something beneficial that will support and encourage the body's natural ability to heal.

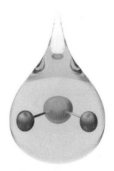

Luckily, the source of that something good is abundant and readily available to everyone. It's water. Water's critical role in a detox is to transport toxins out of cells and then out of the body.

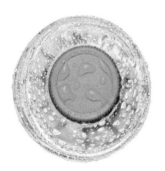

The more well-hydrated you are, the more effectively you will shed toxins. However, even water these days has chemical additives meant to improve taste, sanitize, and alter the "hardness" of the water. To avoid those chemicals, opt for non-treated spring water. You can find spring water at your local grocery store or health food retailer. The next best alternative is to consume water that has been distilled and therefore free of impurities.

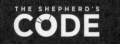

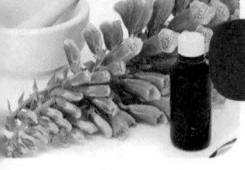

You need only seek out a special water source during the week of your detox. After that, you should return to your water of choice. Since this routine is so accessible and affordable, you may choose to detox on a more regular basis to keep yourself free of cell-damaging chemicals. Keep it to no more than once a month so that your body doesn't become nutrient deficient.

> *Come, everyone who thirsts, come to the waters;*
> *and he who has no money, come, buy and eat!*
> *Come, buy wine and milk without money and without*
> *price. Why do you spend your money for that which*
> *is not bread, and your labor for that which does not*
> *satisfy? Listen diligently to me, and eat what is good,*
> *and delight yourselves in rich food.*
>
> **Isaiah 55:1-2**

Though these words are an allegory for what comes from the fullness of God's power in your life, both drinking water and eating what is good can be the doorways to delight!

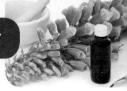

THE TRUTH ABOUT FATS

Balanced nutrition is our first line of defense against the factors that rob us of a long, healthy life. While there is nothing we can do to stop time, we absolutely can fend off disease and suffering. We do that primarily through a lifestyle that includes physical fitness fueled by energy found in foods that are part of a ketogenic diet.

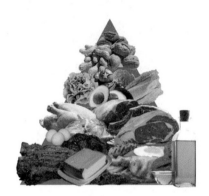

The ketogenic diet replaces such things as chemical additives, refined sugars, and highly processed foods with the healthy fats our bodies need. The ketogenic diet avoids harmful foods that lead to oxidation throughout the organs and body systems we rely on.

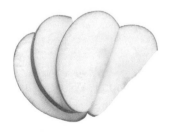

Oxidation is what causes rust on a car or the browning of a sliced apple. The result of oxidation on the human body is, in effect, deterioration along with the release of free radicals. Very nasty. Free radicals are unstable molecules that further damage cells or even alter normal cells and attack our DNA. That's not a battle we can fight while feeding our bodies with junk food!

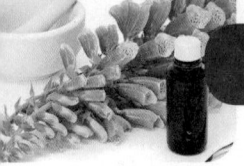

Fast foods and both highly refined and processed foods actually lead to nutritional deficiencies that contribute to oxidative stress. The outward signs of a body attacked by oxidative stress include:

Gray hair

Fatigue

Joint pain

Weakened immune system

Memory loss

Fear not, there's no need for despair! We now understand the blueprint for a diet that can actually reduce your exposure to toxins while rejuvenating the body from within. Forget the lies!

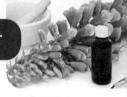

My soul will be satisfied as with fat and rich food, and my mouth will praise you with joyful lips,

Psalm 63:5

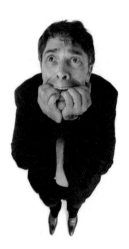

Fat and rich foods are not to be feared! What began as a low-fat "supposed" health craze has indeed led to a nation of low-fat consumers with a dangerous increase in oxidative stress. We've been afraid of the very fats that are a satiating, energy giving, and tasty part of a balanced diet. These smart fat options include nuts, olive and coconut oils, and avocados, among others. These are delicious and appropriate substitutions for diets high in carbs like pasta, potatoes, and pastries.

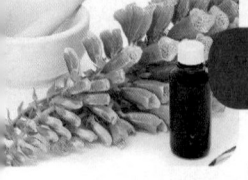

The healing source of energy comes from natural ketones derived from the normal metabolism of fat. Once ketones become our fuel source rather than complex carbohydrates, our organs begin to function at their best. Our skin becomes more resilient and supple. Our kidneys purify our body more easily and thoroughly. We become a much more efficient and lively machine! With this single body meant to last us a lifetime, it's ultimately important to put only the best in if we want to bring the best out.

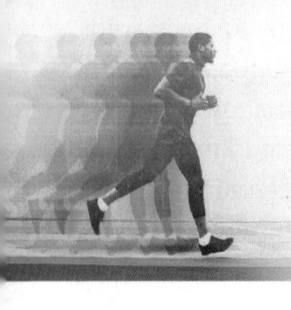

Getting into a state of ketosis allows your body to put energy into the finer things in life--like aging gracefully, with gladness and a feeling of well being. How about longevity? Indeed, promoting optimal bodily functioning typically results in a longer and more comfortable life.

A longer life may sound daunting. These days it is common for disease and illness to wreak havoc even early in life. Most frequently to those living with poor diet and lifestyle choices. Fortunately, research shows following a ketogenic diet can be protection against such a fate.

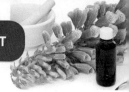

KETOSIS AND AGE-RELATED DISEASE

Age-related disease has a direct correlation to life expectancy. Therefore, the statistics on ketosis' effects on such illnesses have lead to significant discoveries and major breakthroughs.

These are just some of the ways ketones have shown benefits in lab tests:

Protection against neurotoxicity in brain cells

Positive results in Parkinson's patients

Improved cognition in Alzheimer's patients

Further studies will continue to redefine the usefulness of ketones in warding off a decline in advanced age.

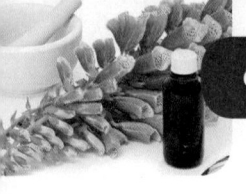

A LOW-CARB LONG LIFE

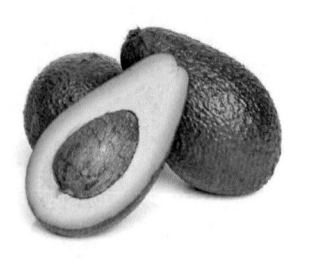

Supporting health with a diet rich in nutrients, antioxidants, high-quality proteins, and healthy fats, while also low in carbs is considered essential. The whole-food qualities characteristic of the ketogenic diet provide the very benefits that alleviate conditions associated with a diet lacking quality. These conditions are common in our society and include those such as obesity, diabetes, and the silent killer, heart disease. Celebrating birthdays without health concerns is a sure way to achieve much happier golden years!

The eyes of all look to you,
and you give them their food in due season.
You open your hand;
you satisfy the desire of every living thing.

Psalm 145:15-16

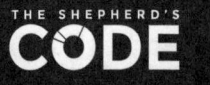

This scripture proves that our desires are within reach! There is no dollar amount or prescription needed for the benefits of what we've been blessed with in our own natural world. We've searched long and hard to find what's been close at hand all along. The puzzle has been fit together beautifully. An astounding variety of bountiful and nutritious resources feeds not only our craving for a satisfied tummy, but the knowledge that we will be well provided for and loved for all time.

ANTI-AGING: THE KETOGENIC DIET VS. THE WESTERN DIET

There is great promise in the link between ketosis and anti-aging. The positive effects on blood sugar, weight, and sustained energy far outweigh the risks of the highly processed foods that line our grocery store shelves. Though many more years of research are needed, it is already obvious that in contrast to the average Western world's diet, the ketogenic option certainly doesn't hurt our chances for longevity.

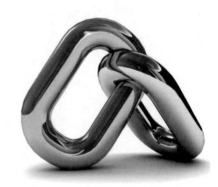

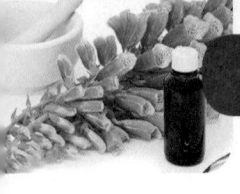

YOU COULD LOOK HALF YOUR AGE

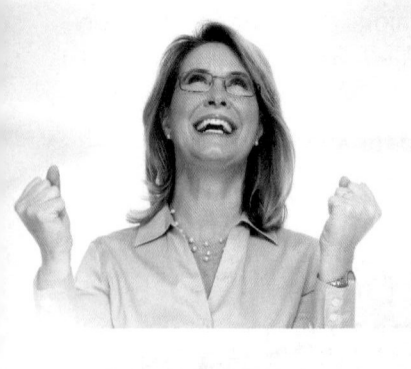

Nothing helps a person stand taller than an unexpected compliment from a stranger. Imagine how frequently celebrities are boosted by compliments by adoring fans, the media, and those marketers wanting to use THEIR face to endorse their products. People really do want to know the celebrity secret to looking Hollywood, and they aren't afraid to ask.

Looking young and vibrant seems mysteriously unattainable, but it's not. The beauty celebrities foster doesn't begin and end with the surface layers of their skin. The results come from a strong and resilient foundation through the layers of their skin. They don't get that from firming creams or exfoliating alone! Instead, they address the layers deep beneath the outer dermis to completely change how their skin reacts to daily stressors and aging.

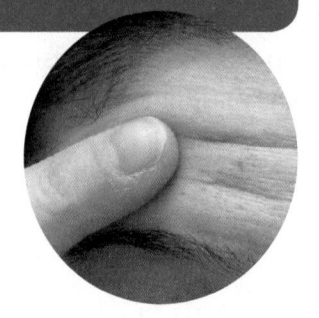

The specific ways the rich and famous nurture their complexion serve to blur the lines when it comes to age.

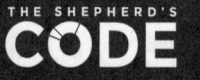

When it's hard to tell which decade a person may be in, there's something besides wrinkles showing on their face. If you think it's the genetic code that determines everything about those looks, think again! Though genetics initially map out the color of our hair, eyes, and skin, it becomes much less an indicator of how our skin will age and react to the exposure of a lifetime.

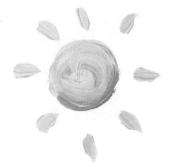

Things such as smoking and sunlight are just two of the biggest offenders we can choose to battle or allow to harm us. Even with an on-point diet, people who consistently absorb harmful rays and adverse chemicals age more rapidly than those who keep themselves protected from such influences.

The stress from chemicals introduced both internally and externally accumulates over time. Unfortunately, this can be seen in the faces of even young people who make choices that degrade their health.

You'll recognize these tell-tale markers as the crows feet and worry lines stretched across even young foreheads! Maybe it's the darkened sun spots appearing where once there was an even skin tone. You better believe there's much more going on just beneath that skin as well.

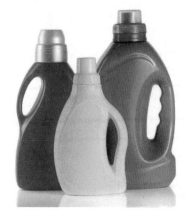

CELEBRITY ANTI-AGING AND WEIGHT LOSS SECRET

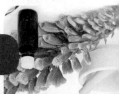

If you are a person who wishes they could turn back the clock to make wiser decisions about your routine expo- sure to chemicals, I'm with you! Most of the population could benefit from these celebrity anti-aging secrets. Getting right to work will mean the results are on their way! While none of us display our years in quite the same way, it is common to notice gravity taking a toll in ways it never did before. Sagging, bagging, and loose- ness partner with wrinkles, spots, and loss of elasticity growing worse until we take action.

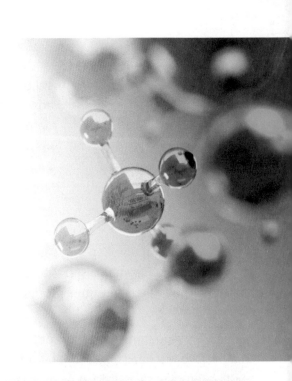

The transformative action of our celebrity anti-aging and weight loss secret ac- tually reverses the sever- ity of all of these signs. It works at the molecular level to repair the damage and symptoms of an ag- ing body and complexion.

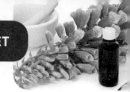

REVERSING THE SIGNS OF AGING

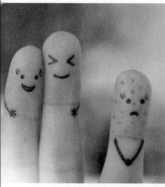

We've all heard it before, "Better late than never." And while it would be wonderful if we had all started on a clean program from day one, it really isn't too late, even if aging has begun to take its toll. Look on the bright side, redness, blemishes, uneven skin tone, and even dryness can be considered the signs that give us the GO to begin a new and healthier routine ASAP.

Don't get down on yourself if you never realized what these signs were warning you. The future is bright! Sticking with the steps in this book will make it possible for you to turn back the clock and reveal a younger you each time you look in the mirror. Remember, your skin is an incredible organ that is always shedding the old and revealing the new. Help it along to find that your new is red-carpet beautiful too.

Fads and temporary fixes are rarely enough to combat what has taken years to fall into disrepair. Diets and healthy routines are best accepted as a lifestyle change instead. The good news is that It can be easy to adjust to these methods that begin rewarding you from the start. This is one lifestyle change that will have the compliments piling up, the pounds falling away, and your body functioning at a higher level than ever before.

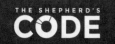

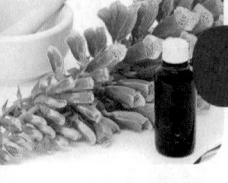

Taking these action steps will put off the aging process, or at least slow it down to a crawl. Correctly applying the techniques in this book will put a focus on bolstering new cell growth. In this way, lackluster skin that has endured stress and the unraveling effects of daily exposure to environmental toxins can begin rejuvenation. Your fresh face will glow with a natural and luminous blush.

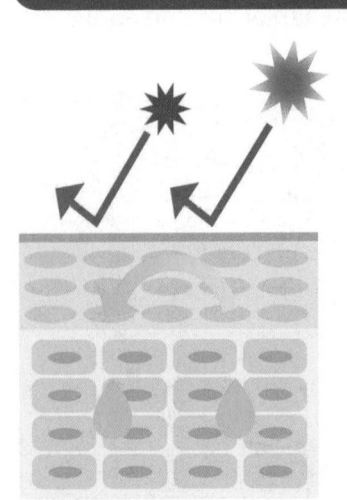

The body, and every organ that is a part of it, heals when wounded and works to support life. Your skin is one of those organs that bear the brunt of both external and internal factors all the time. For your largest organ to remain an effective barrier to the outside world it too must heal and fight to stay as young as possible. As soon as excessive dryness or weakness due to lost elasticity become the norm, your skin is no longer as able to protect you or heal from whatever comes its way.

As if that alone weren't problem enough, failing skin actually puts all the rest of your body in danger. A body without protective layers of skin simply wouldn't survive. Luckily, as we bolster the structure and foundation of our skin, we strengthen our overall defenses and begin to reverse the signs of aging.

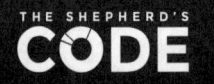

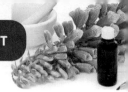

WHY NEVER WASHING YOUR FACE REALLY IS OKAY

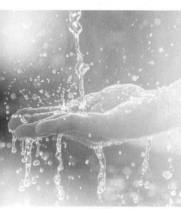

Would you believe that washing your face is the very first thing that's wrong with your current skincare regimen? It's true! As a culture, we have bought into the belief that cleanliness means being sterile. Our bodies are not meant to be sterile! The billions of beneficial bacteria that we coexist with are hugely supportive of the healthy balance we ultimately want to achieve.

That means it's okay to have a bit of "dirt" on our skin. In fact, most people may actually respond negatively to anything more than the use of a gentle cleanser more than once a week. Washing strips away the protective oils and even dead skin cells that keep underlying layers safe. When these are removed toxins have an open door to get in and accelerate the real dirty work we want to put a stop to.

Once you begin the cycle of chemical warfare to try to achieve a camera-ready face, it takes more and longer to get there. These days we battle skin issues our grandparents never even thought about.

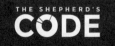

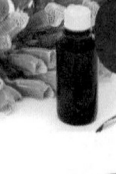

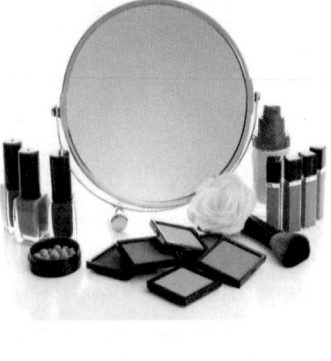

Sure, the generation of celebrities who first graced the screen wore a little makeup, but they were gorgeous even without. And now, with super-high-definition cameras, celebrities just can't afford to look caked with makeup. The Celebrity Anti-aging and Weight-loss Secret has nothing to do with quick-fix-products full of promises.

All it takes is a clean towel and a little lukewarm water. A gentle wipe down does wonders for freshening up and maintaining the natural pH balance your skin prefers. This, along with the techniques in this book, is all you need to find that perfect balance and correct the issues that cause damage and rob you of the flawless skin waiting beneath the surface.

THE ONLY SKIN CARE PRODUCT YOU WILL EVER NEED

Today you've learned how to purify your skin from the inside out. You know how to detox from chemicals and how to eat a diet high in healthy fats for healing and sustenance. There is one last thing that puts the finishing touches on glowing skin. It takes what's already radiant and makes it fully luminous.

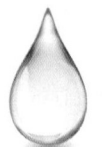

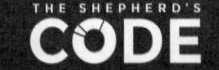

Not only will this give you the compliments you've been waiting for, but it will protect your skin so that you retain that fresh and supple complexion. The barely noticeable sheen will reflect natural light in a way that makes you look like nature's very own gift from above.

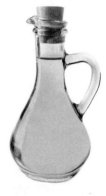

Are you curious about what can have such an incredible effect? It's simple, it's natural, and it's even quite inexpensive! It's oil. Are you surprised? We've been trained to think that oil is something to steer clear of and to remove from our faces at any expense. Well, this isn't just any oil I'm talking about.

Certain oils serve to nourish and protect delicate skin. Without enough of the natural oils our body makes, we may become dry and flaky looking. Too much of it may clog pores and lead to irritation. Wash away too much of it and your body will respond by overproducing to make up for it.

It's challenging to keep on top of because day by day our needs change according to our activity level and the climate.

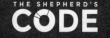

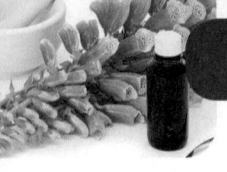

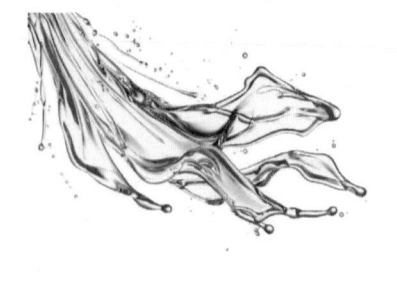

One spot flaky, one spot oily. It can be frustrating, but it's not at all a reason to completely discount the benefits of oil for your face. Using an oil after a gentle cleansing with water tells your skin it is both clean and protected. Instead of putting energy into replacing stripped oils, it can feed and restore the living tissues below.

Once you find the best oil for your skin type, you will be amazed at how the results outperform the entire arsenal of lotions, creams, and treatments you've been slaving over for years. The high-quality oils we want you to enjoy are hypoallergenic, affordable, and perfect for all skin types.

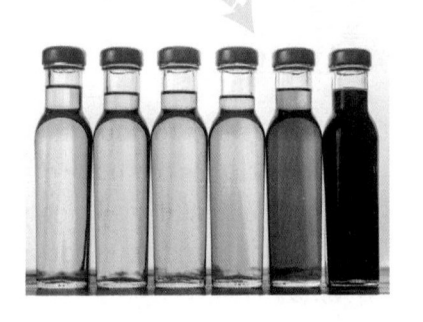

THE FLAWLESS FINISH

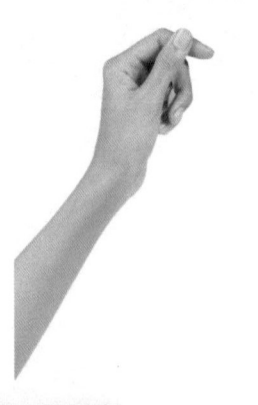

Your flawless finish will come by trial and error. Following your detox, you will assess your skin week to week to identify what it's telling you. You can choose an oil treatment according to your skin's conditions that week. If you are unsatisfied with the results, feel free to detox again and redirect your course using a different oil.

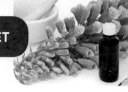

For dry skin:

Dry skin is more susceptible to fine lines and wrinkles. Moringa oil will plump the skin and fill lines with a matte finish. Just two drops daily will provide the intense moisture and antioxidants dry patches need to heal.

For oily skin:

Pull impurities and blockages from your pores using Monoli oil (or Argan oil). Its anti-aging properties are ideal for inflamed or irritated skin. A few drops of oil used once a day after washing will treat and heal.

For combination skin:

Meadowsea Foam or cold-pressed extra-virgin olive oil can be used in combination with other oils for both oily or dry skin. You will come away from this treatment with a more pure, youthful, and even skin tone. Apply these oils twice daily until your complexion is glowing. Then apply just once every evening.

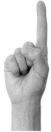

If any one of these oils does not work for your complexion at first, do the one-week detox and try a different option. Within a few weeks, you will have found the oil that works best for you.

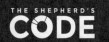

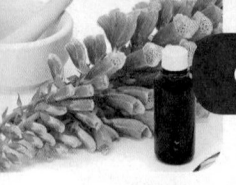

Keep healthy and hydrated with a smile on your face! You are beautiful! Then go forth with a confidence and faith that shows from the inside out. You have the wisdom of Truth, the willing guidance of God whenever you need it, and a bright future of promise.

Have nothing to do with irreverent, silly myths. Rather train yourself for godliness; for while bodily training is of some value, godliness is of value in every way, as it holds promise for the present life and also for the life to come. The saying is trustworthy and deserving of full acceptance.

1Timothy 4:7-9

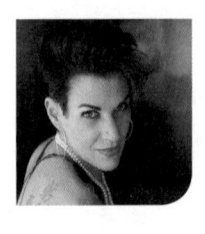

All things are possible!

Kristina Wilds

HEALTHY BRAIN MANUAL

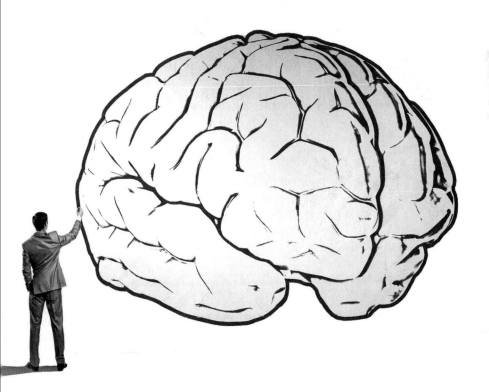

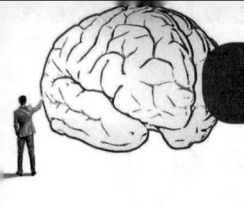

The contents of this document are based upon my opinions of *The Shepherd's Code* unless otherwise noted. This work is intended to share knowledge and information learned through research, experience, and discussions with others. The opinions of others, such as in the comments and the forum, are their own and are not endorsed by *The Shepherd's Code*. The information contained herein is not intended to diagnose, treat, cure or prevent any condition or disease, but rather to provide general information that is intended to be used for educational purposes only. Please consult with your physician or healthcare practitioner if you have any concerns. By using, viewing and interacting with *The Shepherd's Code* or **shepherdscode.com** website, you agree to all terms of engagement, thus assuming complete responsibility for your own actions. The authors and publishers will not claim accountability, nor shall they be held liable for any loss or injury sustained by you. Use, view and interact with these resources at your own risk. All products and information given to you by *The Shepherd's Code* and its related companies are strictly for informational purposes only. While every attempt has been made to verify the accuracy of information provided on our website and within our publications, neither the authors nor the publishers are responsible for assuming liability for possible inaccuracies. The authors and publishers disclaim any responsibility for the inaccuracy of the content, including but not limited to errors or omissions. Loss of property, injury to self or others, and even death could occur as a direct or indirect consequence of the use and application of any content found herein. Please act responsibly. The information provided may need to be downloaded and/or viewed using third party software, such as Acrobat. It's the user's responsibility to install the software necessary to view such information. Any downloads, whether purchased or given for free from our website, related websites or hosting systems are performed at the user's own risk. Although we take great preventative measures, we cannot warranty that our websites are free of corrupting computer codes, viruses or worms. If you are a minor, you can use this service only with permission and guidance from your parents or guardians.

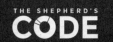

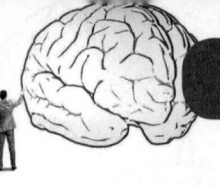

Dealing with memory loss
is a terrible and trying experience,

both for the person who is suffering from it, and for all the people that surround them. It can range from little annoyances and reduced quality of living to the devastation of watching someone we love quietly waste away. Knowing the Lord is in control provides some comfort but doesn't change the fact that the failure of a loved ones' mind is a difficult change to adapt to.

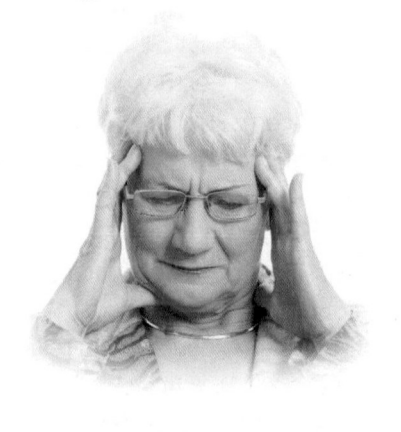

To make matters worse, for most of the diseases and afflictions that cause such effects, there has been no cure, and therapy has had limited success... but that's all changing. There are some steps we can take to potentially prevent such terrible things from happening or at least to slow down the effects in severe cases. It is so comforting to know that we are not alone in our struggles and there are ways to help it all go more smoothly.

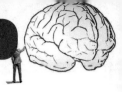

Behold, I will bring to it health and healing, and I will heal them and reveal to them abundance of prosperity and security.

Jeremiah 33:6

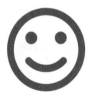

In this report, we will first take a look at how our memory works and what are some of the most common causes of memory loss in human adults. Following that, we will see how switching from a diet loaded with carbohydrates to one high in "healing fats" can help reduce memory loss, and how we can potentially repair our memory.

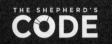

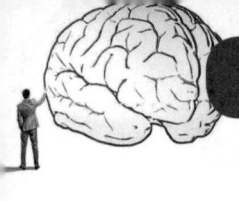
HOW OUR MEMORY WORKS

Our memory is a tricky thing.

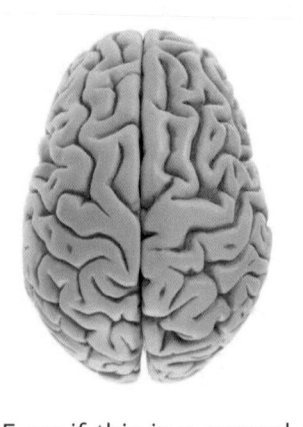

As our memory becomes weaker we find we forget things as simple as where we left our keys to bigger things like dentist appointments and the story of our past.

Even if this is a normal process in itself, there is a lot we can do to slow it down, or even prevent it to some extent. After all, not all people suffer from dementia and other terrible afflictions, and some people retain more mental clarity in their twilight years than others.

As we age, our lives seem to go by faster, and we seem to remember things **less and less**. Well, even if this might be inevitable, there are certain factors that have been linked to this.

Before we explore these things that affect our memory negatively, it could be useful to try and understand the basics of how our memory works. What does it really mean to "forget"?

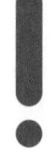 There are three key processes which we undergo when we form new memories. First, our sensory apertures (eyes, ears, hands, etc.) have to perceive something. Then, the impression that we gained from this observation is stored in our short

 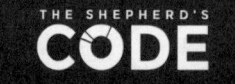

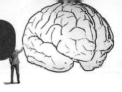

term memory, where it can stay for around 20 to 30 seconds. After that, it is either discarded or committed to our long-term memory, where it can stay indefinitely.

We can remember about 7 items at a time for about half a minute.

Our **short term memory** serves as a buffer, so that we don't get overwhelmed with information. It can typically store around 7 different items at a time for about half a minute. That's why we sometimes hear a 10-digit number and we almost instantly forget it. Now, there are tricks (like clustering) that we do in order to increase the density of information in our short term memory. If we do not try to remember that phone number as 10 individual digits, but rather as several groups of 2 or 3 digits, it suddenly becomes less of a problem.

This gives us enough time to dial a number and then subsequently forget it—or rather, not remember it. When we want to commit something to memory, we often have to repeat it

`0 123456 789`

`0733956 700`

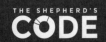

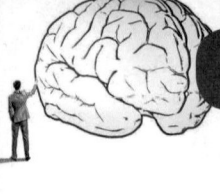

to ourselves. Because transfer from **short-term to long-term** memory happens gradually, and sometimes it takes more time than the 20-30 seconds, we have to "refresh" our short-term memory by repeating the information. Of course, when the experience is important to us or has a powerful or unexpected effect, it takes much less time to remember it.

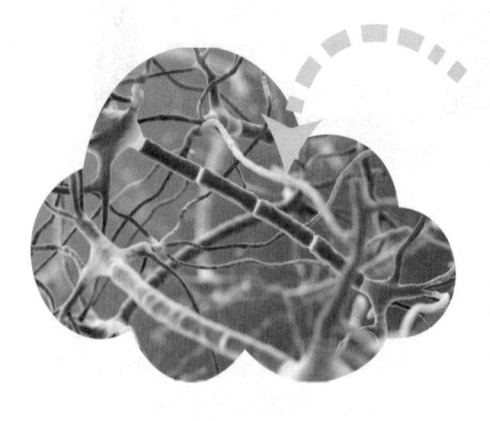

Now, our brain consists of billions of **individual neurons**, but our memory as such is not a specific set of neurons in one part of our brain. When we think of shoes, the word is stored in one area, the concept itself in the other, how they look in the third, and the sound they make in the fourth part of our brain.

All of this information is simultaneously pulled when we try to recall it, and we remember the complete object with no sweat. Neurons themselves are not where our memory is stored; it is actually in the connections between different neurons, called **synapses**.

These synapses are **pathways** down which electric impulses go in order for neurons to communicate with each other. If there is an electric impulse down one pathway more often than down the other, the first pathway, or synapse, gets stronger.

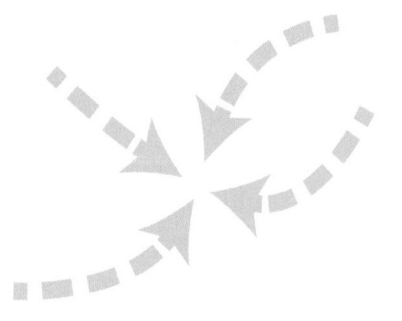

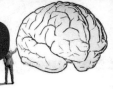

When we learn new information, it creates a number of **new connections** between neurons in our brain. If we use and reuse this information, that particular connection grows stronger, and we can remember that particular thing more effectively.

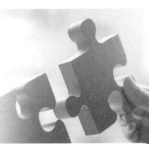

If you think of any **skill**, this is how we learn it. We practice the same pattern, movement, or sequence over and over, until we have mastered it. In our brain, certain neurons made connections all over the brain, and as we repeated the sentence, the movement, equation, musical passage, or whatever else, we strengthened these connections.

When we do not use certain synapses, their strength over time fades. This is why it gets harder and harder to recall certain information after a long period of time. Bear in mind that not all the synapses connected to a particular memory would decay at the same rate.

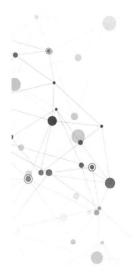

Forgetting, simply put, is the inability to retrieve information.

Now, this can happen for more than one **reason**. Obviously, that particular brain path might be damaged (or sufficiently weakened—memory itself is there, but we can't physically access it).

You might have experienced a terrible psychological trauma at some point in your life and have repressed memories. In this case, nothing

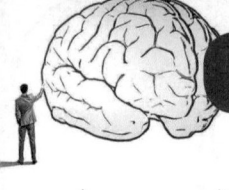
is wrong with your memory in itself, but you have put psychological locks to protect yourself from remembering because it is too painful.

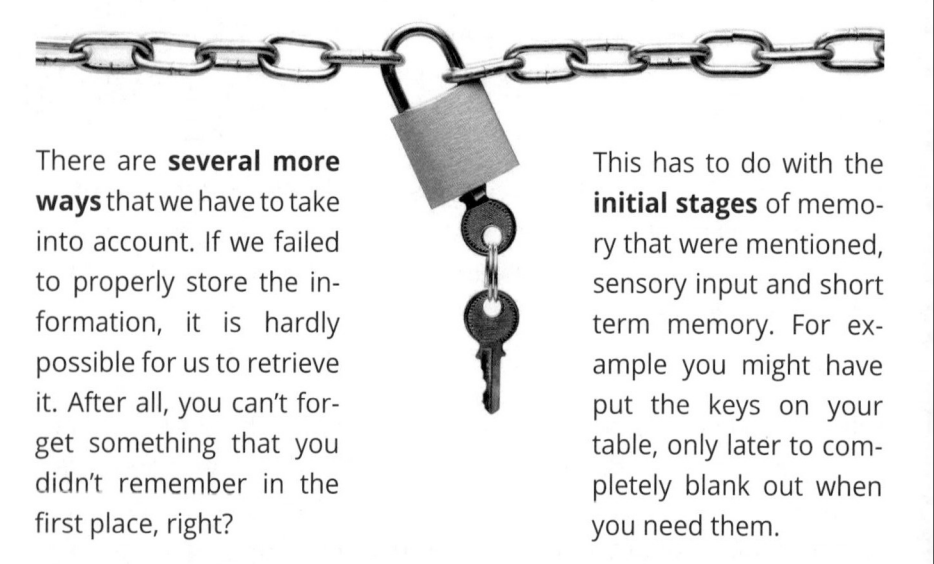

There are **several more ways** that we have to take into account. If we failed to properly store the information, it is hardly possible for us to retrieve it. After all, you can't forget something that you didn't remember in the first place, right?

This has to do with the **initial stages** of memory that were mentioned, sensory input and short term memory. For example you might have put the keys on your table, only later to completely blank out when you need them.

What if you didn't even **register** where you put them?

Sometimes you can be **distracted** by either something going on (cell phone), or by your inner train of thought. You put the keys on the table automatically and simply didn't even register it. This would be failure at a sensory level.

Likewise, you might have paid attention to where you put the keys at the moment, but you simply **didn't bother** to move that information from your short term to your long term memory. These situations often happen when we are absent minded.

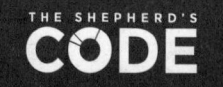

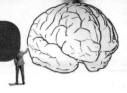

WHAT CAUSES MEMORY LOSS?

 Medication

A whole slew of different medicines can cause memory impairment. Anti-anxiety meds, antihistamines (anti-allergy), antidepressants, muscle relaxants, sleeping pills, pain meds, and tranquilizers are only some of the possible culprits. This is not only limited to prescription drugs, so always be sure to check the negative side effects, especially if you're taking over-the-count-

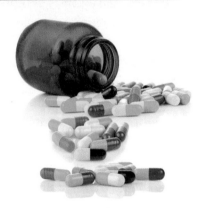

er medicine. If you're not certain about the side-effects, be sure to consult with your doctor or a specialist before you start your therapy.

A huge benefit of adopting *The Shepherd's Code* lifestyle is an opportunity to be taken off your meds by your doctor. We have hundreds of life changing testimonials proving this is possible.

 Head injury

Physical trauma can lead to lesions, blood clots, inflammation, and other types of damage in our brain. This is the most straightforward type of brain damage, and it can be extremely dangerous. Heavy, or multiple, concussions can have terrible consequences on mental health.

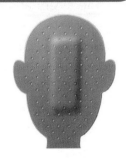

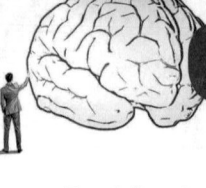
Danish scientists have found that concussions and skull fractures can increase the risk of developing **mental disorders** by more than 400%. Contact sports like hockey or American football have shown that players often end up with depression, anxiety, pill addictions, alcoholism, migraines, and all sorts of other issues that greatly decrease their quality of life, sometimes even leading to suicide.

 Stroke

One of the top five leading causes of death in the US, stroke is a disease in which arteries that supply blood to the brain can't do the job properly. Our brains are supplied with **blood** from a large number of small blood vessels that branch out from main blood arteries that go to our brain. If blood clots are formed or a blood vessel ruptures, stroke occurs.

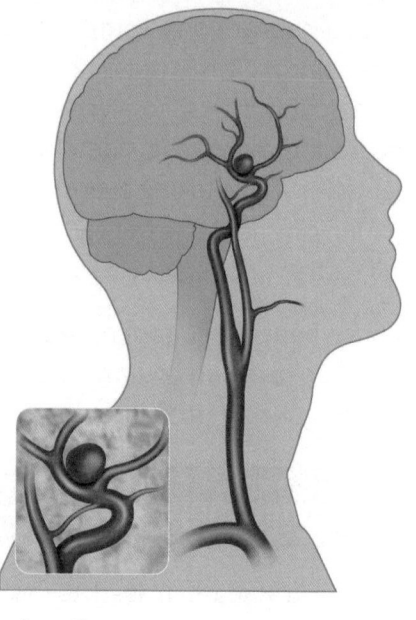

When a **blood clot** is formed, it clogs the artery and reduces or completely stops the blood flow to the brain. If it bursts, all the blood spills out and nothing gets to where it's supposed to go. When an area of the brain that should be supplied by damaged blood vessel doesn't receive enough blood, it also doesn't get oxygen and nutrients that are necessary for it to function. When this happens, brain cells stop functioning, and start to die out.

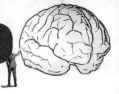

😞 Dementia

Dementia is a category of brain diseases that causes progressive loss of mental abilities and memory in people who suffer from it. **Neurodegenerative diseases** cause shrinking of brain mass and death of brain cells, and typically they get worse as time goes by. Since these diseases physi-

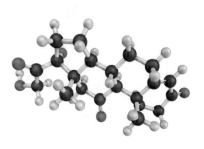

cally alter brain structure, the effects are irreversible, and often untreatable. Again, fortunately the medical community has been studying the ketogenic diet for some time, and it's been proven that a high "healing fat" diet can slow or stop dementia at all stages.

😞 Sleep Deprivation

Very few things can have as bad an effect on our health as chronic sleep deprivation. No matter if it's caused by insomnia, bad sleeping habits, sleep disorders, or a punishing daily schedule due to various circumstances, sleep deprivation

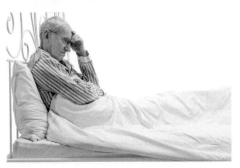

has an adverse effect on both our **physical and mental health.**

In respect to our memory, insufficient sleep leads to attention deficit and inability to quickly recall information. Since our attention suffers

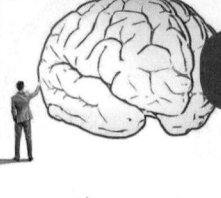
the most, we can experience memory lapses in our short term memory, such as omitting words while speaking or taking down notes. But we can also have the same problem with previously learned information, like forgetting to add crucial ingredients while cooking.

When a person is **severely sleep deprived**, their mental performance suffers, and in worst case scenarios, it can lead to accidents, injuries, or death.

 Stress

Stress has a **multitude** of negative effects on our wellbeing, but it also affects our ability to concentrate. If we are distracted, it is less likely that we will be able to commit something to memory, leading to "encoding failure"–the memory hasn't been stored in the first place, so there is nothing to recall at a later date.

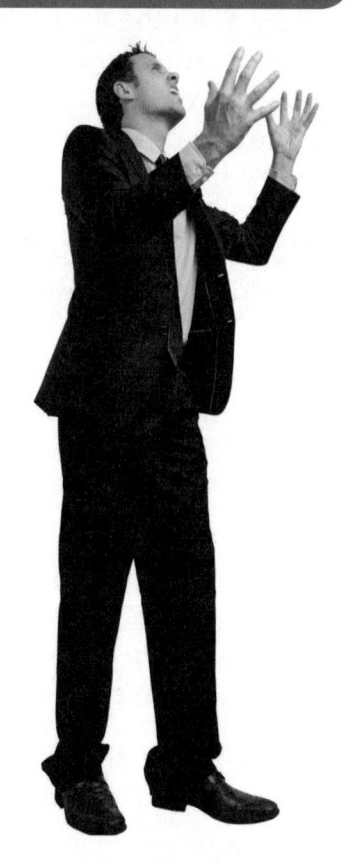

In addition, it has been established that stress is one of the factors that lead to various mental disorders, such as depression and anxiety which negatively influence our ability to focus and remember things. To make matters worse, recent studies have found a potential connection between stress and progression of **Alzheimer's** in certain patients.

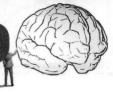

Bad Diet

If your diet **isn't balanced properly**, there could be vitamin or mineral deficiencies that could in turn cause significant brain damage over time. Deficiency of vitamins B1 and B12 specifically, has been shown to lead to increased deterioration of our brain structure.

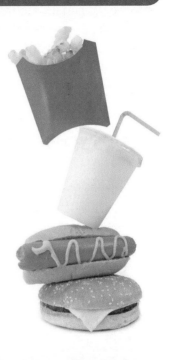

In addition, clogged arteries can lead to a **reduced blood flow** to the brain. This in turn would lead to oxygen starvation in select areas. The effect is similar to having a lot of mini-strokes; the damage of such an event is negligible on its own, but it accumulates over time, and can be as bad as a full-on stroke.

Disease and Medical Conditions

A number of viruses, bacteria, and fungi can also be **extremely harmful** to our brains, particularly the ones that attack our immune or nervous systems. HIV, syphilis, meningitis, and a plethora of other microorganisms can all do considerable brain damage and cause memory loss.

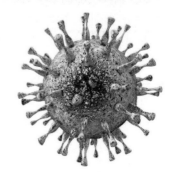

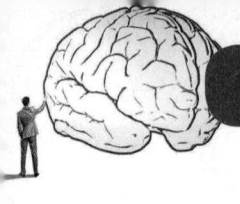

Diabetes, high blood pressure, and other types of **chronic conditions** can also have a negative effect on your memory. This is mostly due to reduced oxygen flow to the brain, or too much sugar in the body.

Last, but not least, things that we consume for **our pleasure and entertainment** have adverse effects on our health as well.

ALCOHOL, DRUGS, AND TOBACCO

Beloved, I urge you as sojourners and exiles to abstain from the passions of the flesh, which wage war against your soul.

1 Peter 2:11

While it is common knowledge that alcohol, drugs, and cigarettes have a damaging effect on our health, the thing that is less clear to most people is why it is so. The effects of alcohol are particularly murky in this area, as there are a large number of seemingly contradictory studies that come out every year.

 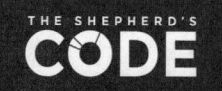

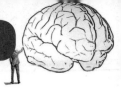

In short, alcohol is purported to be healthy when **consumed in small doses** (a glass of wine or two), but is very unhealthy when drunk in larger quantities.

Even if you're not a regular heavy drinker, drinking more than five drinks in one day has been linked to increased likelihood of cancer.

What are the effects on our mental health?

Alcohol alters our brain chemistry **in two ways:**

1 It acts as a **depressant** by affecting certain **neurotransmitters**. Neurotransmitters are chemical messengers that are the basis of how neurons in our body and brain communicate. Alcohol increases activity of **GABA**, a neurotransmitter that slows down brain activity, and hinders the activity of glutamate, another neurotransmitter that does the opposite.

In turn, this makes us sluggish, slurs our speech, and lowers our inhibitions.

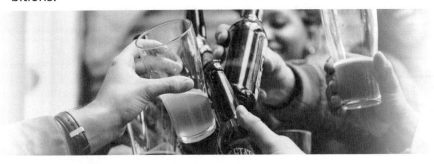

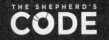

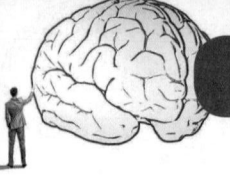

2

Alcohol **increases** production of the hormone called **dopamine.**

Dopamine is part of our **reward system**, and it is what makes us feel good when we drink. Due to increased dopamine production, we often want to drink more, and sometimes end up addicted.

As we consume alcohol over time, our **tolerance grows** and dopamine production becomes lower and lower. Even when we stop experiencing the dopamine high, the habit has been formed, and alcohol addiction remains.

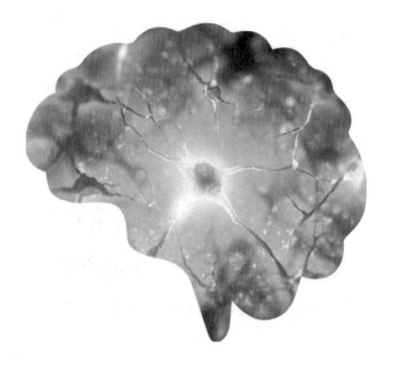

Physically, alcohol **destroys brain cells** in certain areas and causes our brains to **shrink** in volume if consumed regularly at high doses. As the end result, prolonged heavy use of alcohol can lead to a debilitating disease called Wernicke–Korsakoff Syndrome which is a kind of dementia, and the effects are irreversible if not treated immediately.

Due to alcohol's effect on our brain chemistry, synapses, and cells, it can also play a role in the onset of other types of **neurodegenerative diseases**, such as Alzheimer's, Parkinson's, and so on.

In summary, alcohol in **small daily doses** can have a protective effect on your health, but if you're a life-long abstainer, you shouldn't start drinking just for the sake of it.

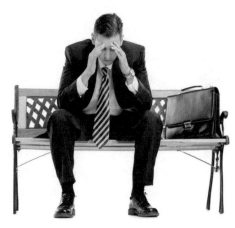

Obviously, alcohol consumption is **not the only unhealthy habit** that should be addressed. Until a few years ago, smoking was a number one cause of preventable deaths in the US. Nicotine is the substance that causes addiction, but it is not as damaging to our health as other substances found in tobacco, such as tar, or heavy metals.

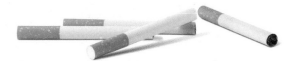

Cigarettes are responsible for a huge number of health issues, from lung cancer, other types of cancer, miscarriages, erectile dysfunction, heart attack, stroke, and the list goes on. Smoking also reduces the amount of oxygen that gets to your brain. In turn, this reduces your mental performance, and it has an adverse effect on memory formation.

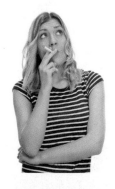

Several studies have shown that people who smoke have **more issues with remembering faces** than non-smokers. In addition, one study found that the amount of nicotine consumed can be linked to poorer recall. When given a memory test, non-smokers did better than light smokers, and light smokers did better than heavy smokers.

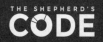

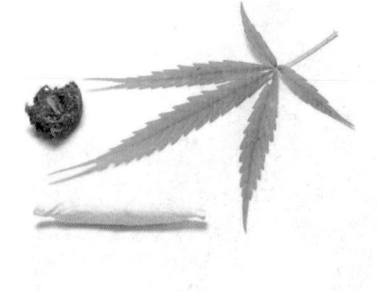

Drugs, particularly synthetic drugs, alter our brain chemistry in an even more extreme manner than tobacco and alcohol, and are thus much more damaging to our brains.

Marijuana, however, has been shown to have real positive medicinal properties, so the leading consensus among health experts is that it can be healthy when used in moderation, similar to drinking a glass of red wine a day.

EFFECTS OF SUGAR ON YOUR MOOD

Even though we think that sugar makes us **feel more energetic** and happy, there is solid evidence to the contrary. A fairly high number of studies done by researchers from various universities and institutes have found links between increased sugar intake and various mental issues. Depression, memory impairment, and mood swings can all be attributed to prolonged overconsumption of sugar in some cases.

For example, in **one study done by Boston University School of Medicine**, over 4,200 people have been periodically tested for their memory and cognition, and researchers also did MRI scans of their brains to measure if there were any changes in volume.

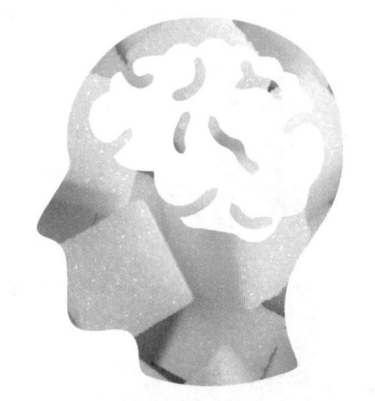

The study found that people who were consuming a lot of soft or sweetened

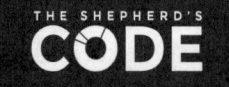

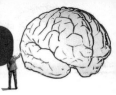

drinks had reduced brain volume and **poorer memory** than the people who didn't drink such drinks.

Based on their results, authors of the study estimated that the difference in brain age can be significant in people from two groups of the same age. Specifically, they found that the brains of people who consume a lot of soft drinks can be 1.5–2.6 years older in terms of total brain volume, and an even more worrying 3.5–13 years older when it comes to memory.

> Furthermore, all of the characteristics found in these cases are consistent with patterns found in people that are vulnerable to Alzheimer's disease.

Several studies have also found links between sugar and various mental disorders that are growing increasingly common in the modern world. One recent study has found that sugar can increase the intensity and add to frequency and intensity of panic and anxiety attacks.

Heavy consumption of sugar has also been tied to depression. One large study done in England, called the Whitehall study, focused on various effects on mortality over a span of 22 years in more than 10,000 people. While it wasn't the main point of the study, researchers also found that men who consumed more than 67 grams of

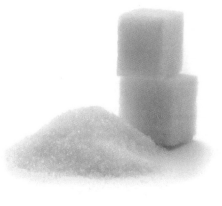

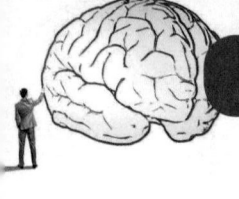
sugar per day were 23% more likely to suffer from depression than men who ate less than 40 grams per day.

Sugar has also been linked to cellular **inflammation and weakening of the immune system**, both of which are known culprits.

> While all of these studies can't be considered as conclusive proof, it is almost certain that **overconsumption of sugar is bad** for our mental health, in addition to already proven negative effects on our physical health.

IMPROVED MENTAL PERFORMANCE ON A KETOGENIC DIET

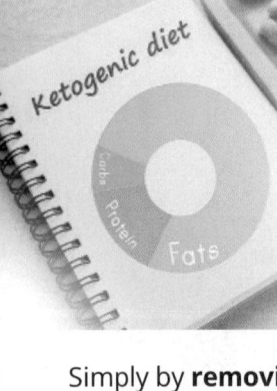

The ketogenic diet has been known to **positively affect** mental conditions, and it has been used as treatment for epilepsy for almost a century.

As ketone bodies replace glucose as a primary source of **fuel for our brain**, a lot of people experience higher thought clarity, better decision making, and some even have feelings of euphoria.

Simply by **removing excess sugar** from your body, you can greatly improve your mental performance and prevent further memory loss. Our bodies have not been designed to eat so much sugar and saturated fats, both commonly found in modern junk food and high carb diets.

 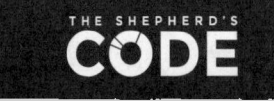

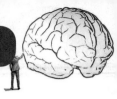

Not only do these sweet and starchy foods **lead to obesity** and unhealthy belly fat, they also have very negative effects on our brains. As previously stated, sugar can lead to mood swings, depression, and anxiety.

Bad diet in general can lead to **mild cognitive impairment**, dementia, stroke, and other afflictions that plague modern society. Just to remind you, we are solely talking about negative effects of sugar-based diets on your mental health—there is a plethora of other types of problems that arise when we talk about our physical health, not the least of which is **diabetes**.

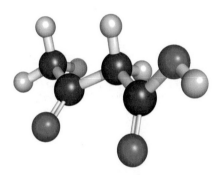

When you stick to you ketogenic diet, you enter **ketosis** and your brain uses ketone bodies as fuel instead of glucose. This rebalances the organism, our insulin levels go back to normal, cellular inflammation is reduced, and we start **burning fat instead of carbohydrates**.

This means that we can also **burn visceral fat** that is responsible for clogging the arteries, and other health issues. The effectiveness of this rebalancing of our organisms is so great that there are some signs that the ketogenic diet has been shown to treat, or at least reduce the symptoms of, neurodegenerative diseases like Alzheimer's, ALS, Parkinson's, and others.

You can have these effects with a normal low carb diet as well, but the effectiveness is much greater if you go full keto, and limit yourself

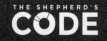

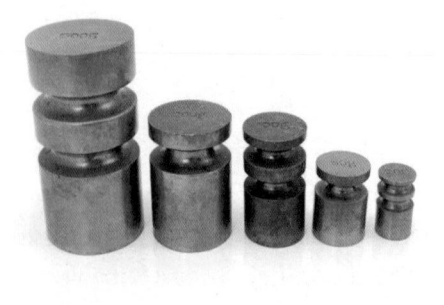

to less than **20 grams of carbs per day**. If you're worried about not having enough sugar in your body, a recent report by the US Institute of Medicine's Food and Nutrition Board states that we need zero grams of carbohydrates in order to survive.

Our liver metabolizes all the **necessary glucose from fats** on a keto diet, so that is not a problem. With that said, it is not advised to eat zero carbs per day, simply because you eliminate a lot of healthy foods from your diet that way.

CAN WE REPAIR OUR MEMORY?

But the Helper, the Holy Spirit, whom the Father will send in my name, he will teach you all things and bring to your remembrance all that I have said to you.

John 14:26

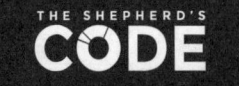

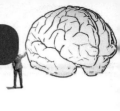

In order **to try and repair** or prevent memory loss, we first need to find its cause. If you find that you (or a person close to you) is becoming increasingly forgetful, agitated, and seem to have memory problems that interfere with your daily life, it is best that you visit your **doctor**.

Your doctor needs to **evaluate the extent of your memory loss** and what the best treatment would be. Typically, he would take a look at your medical history, do a physical exam, and do verbal tests to try and **determine** what is wrong with you.

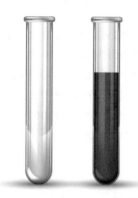

If this is not enough to **determine the problem**, you may have to do urine and blood tests, neurological tests, and maybe even do brain scans such as CAT (computerized axial tomography) or MRI (magnetic resonance imaging) scans.

When the **cause** of your memory loss has been established, a specialist can suggest a **treatment.**

Luckily, this condition is often **reversible**. For example, if your memory loss is caused by medication, moving off those meds and creating alternative therapy could solve the problem.

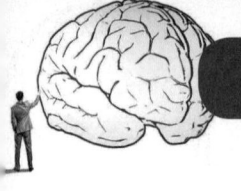
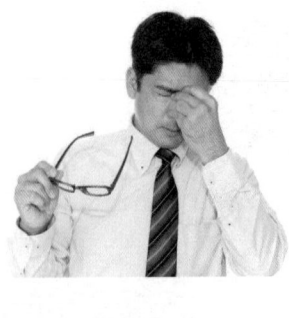

If it's brought on by anxiety, depression, or general stress, your situation can be **improved** if these conditions are addressed. In case of dietary issues, various food supplements can be introduced if diet change is impossible (due to allergies or some other conditions).

When the memory loss is caused due to physical trauma or a stroke, sometimes **physical therapy or mental exercises** can help regain functionality–relearning how to walk or tie your shoelaces, for example. In some cases of amnesia, memory comes back on its own, over time.

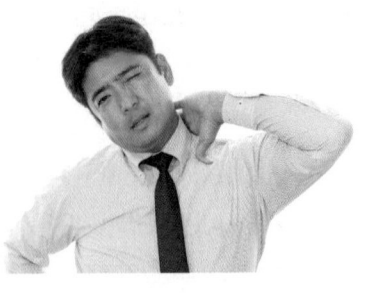

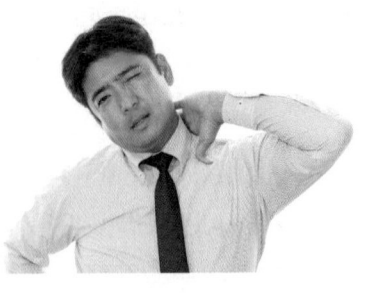

If memory loss is caused by an **underlying condition** such as high blood pressure, it could potentially be restored by treating the main problem, typically with appropriate medicine or therapy.

With all that said, there are **certain habits and lifestyle changes** that you can introduce to combat memory loss in general. Whether medical conditions or general aging is in question, certain activities and strategies have been proven to both prevent memory loss and stimulate regrowth of brain cells.

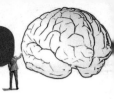

Neurogenesis, or formation of new brain cells, is promoted by a group of genes that are called BDNF (brain derived neurotrophic factor). We know this because MRI scans have shown that this gene pathway is connected to brain cell growth and formation of connections, or synapses, in it.

> *These **changes in your lifestyle** that you should consider implementing are not rocket science, and most of them are **beneficial** to you in other ways as well.*

 Exercise.

Studies have shown that there is a **direct correlation** between physical activity and our brain health.

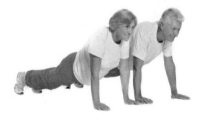

In one year-long study, individuals who engaged in exercise were actually growing and expanding the brain's memory center one to two percent per year, whereas typically that center would have continued to decline in size.

 Reduce overall calorie consumption.

 Reduce carbohydrate consumption.

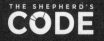

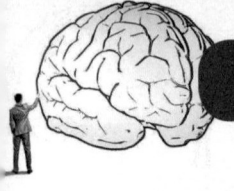
 **Increase healthy fat consumption.**

 **Increase your omega-3 fat intake and reduce the intake of omega-6 fats.**

While both omega-3 and omega-6 fats are good for us, they need to be in a certain ratio. Reduce the consumption of processed vegetable oils, and use more organic olive oil, coconut oil, animal fat, or fish oil in your diet. Krill oil is even better than fish oil as it also contains astaxan-

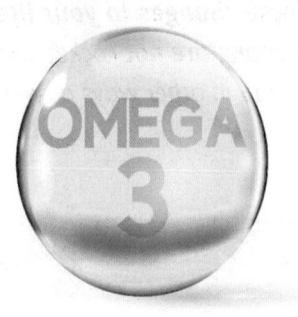

thin, a compound that is good for your brain. It's exactly the new lifestyle *The Shepherd's Code* creates for you.

According to **Dr. Perlmutter**, a renowned neurologist, we can influence our genes in a positive way:

"We interact with our genome every moment of our lives, and we can do so very, very positively," he says. *"Keeping your blood sugar low is very positive in terms of allowing the genes to express reduced inflammation, which increase the production of life-giving antioxidants."* So that's **rule number one**: You can change your genetic destiny.

 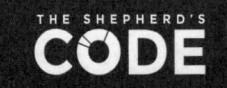

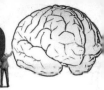

Rule number two:

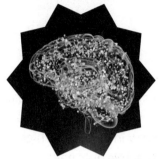

You can change your genetic destiny to **grow new brain cells**, specifically in the hippocampus.... Your brain's memory center regenerates. You are constantly growing new brain cells into your 50s, 60s, 70s, 80s, and 90s (throughout your lifetime) through a process called **neurogenesis**.

That said, these two ideas come together because you can turn on your genes through **lifestyle choices** that enhance neurogenesis and that enhance regrowth of cells and expansion of your brain's memory center. This was **proven** by researchers recently. They demonstrated that there are factors under our control that can make that happen.

As you may have noticed, most of the items on the list can be achieved by **fully switching** to a high healing-fats ketogenic diet. Even so, there are ways that a ketogenic diet can further be adapted to promote memory repair.

This **"dementia diet"** is based on several additional rules, besides the low carb intake of a standard ketogenic diet:

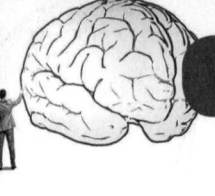
Eliminate all sugar and **sweeteners** (both artificial and natural ones), starchy carbohydrates (bread, pasta, rice, potatoes, and so on) and grains from your diet. Grains are problematic as a lot of people have gluten sensitivity or other sorts of dietary problems without knowing it.

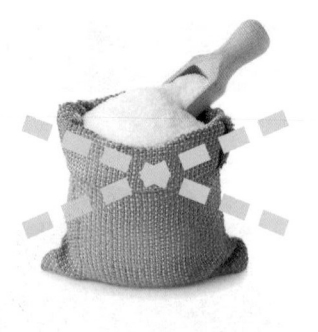

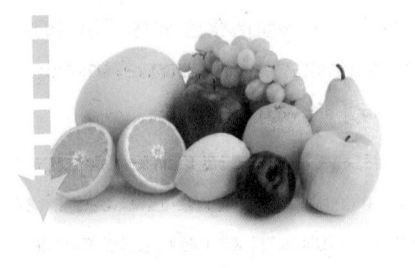

Reduce the amount of **fruit** you eat, and mostly eat berries and nuts— berries are low in sugar and high in antioxidants, while nuts have a lot of minerals and healthy fats in them.

Eat protein from high-quality sources, and avoid **dairy** products. Good sources of protein are grass-fed meats, wild-caught fish, and free range eggs. Dairy is bad for you because it can cause cell inflammation if you are lactose intolerant or sensitive.

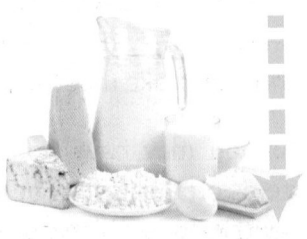

Eat a lot of **non-starchy** vegetables.

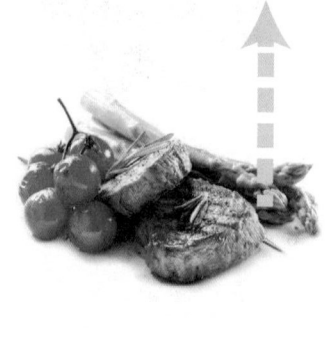

Eat enough **healthy fats** to sustain you. Besides the fats you can find in animal products that are also a source of protein, you should use olive oil, or medium-chain triglyceride (MCT) oil to balance out your omega 3's and omega 6's, as well as gain the best from your keto diet.

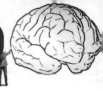

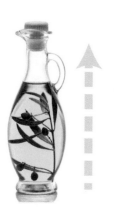

MCT oil is a great addition because it is very easily absorbed by us, and the liver can directly convert it to ketone bodies. The effect of these types of fats is only now being researched more thoroughly, but the results are promising–several studies show that they can have a positive effect on neurodegenerative disorders such as Alzheimer's and Parkinson's.

Our health is **important**. Our memory and our ability to think are what make us human, and we must fight with all our might to keep them with us as long as possible. Luckily for us, it isn't that hard. **Exercise, eat well, sleep well,** and take care of your wellbeing in general, and your body will reward you. Not only will you be happier, but you will also have more energy and less pain, and you will be able to think and experience life with greater clarity than ever.

> *But he said to me, "My grace is sufficient for you, for my power is made perfect in weakness." Therefore I will boast all the more gladly of my weaknesses, so that the power of Christ may rest upon me.*
>
> *2 Corinthians 12:9*

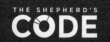

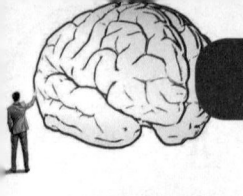

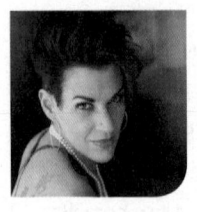

All things are possible!

Kristina Wilds

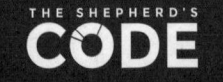